Cultural Fault Lines in Healthcare

Cultural Fault Lines in Healthcare

Reflections on Cultural Competency

Michael C. Brannigan

LEXINGTON BOOKS
Lanham • Boulder • New York • Toronto • Plymouth, UK

Published by Lexington Books
A wholly owned subsidary of The Rowman & Littlefield Publishing Group, Inc.
4501 Forbes Boulevard, Suite 200, Lanham, Maryland 20706
www.lexingtonbooks.com

Estover Road, Plymouth PL6 7PY, United Kingdom

British Library Cataloguing in Publication Information Available

Library of Congress Cataloging-in-Publication Data

Brannigan, Michael C., 1948–
Cultural fault lines in healthcare : reflections on cultural competency / Michael C. Brannigan.
p. cm.
Includes bibliographical references and index.
ISBN 978-0-7391-4966-9 (hardback) — ISBN 978-0-7391-4967-6 (paper) — ISBN 978-0-7391-
4968-3 (ebook)
1. Transcultural medical care—United States. 2. Cultural competence—United States. I. Title.
RA418.5.T73B73 2012
362.1—dc23
2011045096

Printed in the United States of America

To my dear friend and colleague
Dr. John Balint,
physician, teacher, scholar, and healer
who embodies genuine presence
throughout his competent caring and compassion

Contents

WITHDRAWN

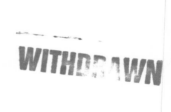

Acknowledgments

In the spirit of this book's underlying theme—to even begin to know the Other, we must first look within ourselves—deep humility accompanies my litany of gratitude to family and friends and to all who have in their own ways taught me this lesson. First, my heartfelt thanks to the staff at Lexington Press for their conscientious support for this project, particularly to Jana Wilson Hodges-Kluck for her remarkable patience, encouragement, and wise guidance, acquisitions assistant Eric Wrona, and Jessica McCleary, production editor, for her marvelous and first-rate work. My appreciation also goes to Diane Brenner for her expert indexing.

I offer my undying gratitude:

To the countless patients who have honored me with the privilege of sharing their intimate moments of suffering, hope, despair, faith, and final peace.

To those physicians, nurses, social workers, hospital staff, clergy, and all professional caregivers who for me have been models of presence and compassion with their patients and patients' families.

To my colleagues at the College of Saint Rose for their unfailing support, particularly Mark Sullivan, Dave Szczerbacki, Father Chris Degiovine, Lorna Shaw, Laura Weed, Dan Thero, and Sr. Rose Regina Smith. Sr. Rose's presence and inspiration are a precious gift of grace.

To my good friend George Pfaff, and in blessed memory of his wife Jane whom I never met personally, but know her grace through George's, for his steadfast commitment to ethics education and moral instruction.

To my colleagues at Alden March Bioethics Institute and Albany Medical College for their dedication to healthcare ethics and their support of my work in intercultural bioethics, particularly to John Balint, Wayne Shelton, Liva Jacoby, Sheila Otto, John Kaplan, Bruce White, Fariah Grant, and Hayley Dittus.

To my colleagues at Cardiff University's Health Communication Research Centre, Srikant Sarangi, Peter Schulz, Per Måseide, Aileen Doyle, Wendy Lewis, and to all those wise students throughout the summer sessions who continue to enrich the pioneering dialogue between communication and ethics in healthcare.

To my Japanese family, friends, and colleagues who continue to teach me invaluable lessons in intercultural sensitivity and understanding, particularly Akira Akabayashi, Kazumasa Hoshino, Tomoaki Tsushida, Kunio and Izumi Aoki, Akio Sakai, and Sachiko and Keiko.

To the many scholars and friends who through their work radiate their dedication to patient well-being and genuine interpersonal rapport between health professionals and patients, especially Ed Pellegrino, Marjorie Sirridge, Marilyn Pesto, Wayne Vaught, Joan Collison, Steve Jeffers, and Landis Downing (now deceased, may Steve and Landis forever live in our hearts), Steve Salanski, Rosemary Flanigan, Rachel Reeder, Ann Grow, Maureen Bryden, Bruce Heckman, Joe Cunneen, and Paul and Eileen Churchill.

And most importantly, to my beloved wife Brooke, for her immeasurable patience, good judgment, keen insights, unfailing encouragement, whose smile lights even the darkest corner, and for whom words are never enough.

To all, I give thanksgiving. May your work in relieving suffering never cease and always keep you strong.

Introduction

*Questioning the ostensibly unquestionable premises of our way of life is argu-
ably the most urgent of the services we owe our fellow humans and ourselves.*—Zygmunt Bauman

This book offers a critical reflection on what it means to be "culturally
competent." At the same time, it is an exercise in thinking out loud, a philosophical prelude to uncover what tends to lie hidden in our encounter with
the patient, the Other, particularly the Other who represents a culture and
worldview seemingly disparate from our own. This is in keeping with philosophy's initial task in revealing what is concealed, as Heidegger reminds us
through the early Greek notions of *aletheia* as "truth" of "unconcealment"
and "nakedness."

What is now surely unhidden in the healthcare domain is that cultural
fault lines exist wherein multiple moral traditions, perspectives, and assumptions are clearly at odds with each other. With our nation comprising at least
66 racial and ethnic groupings, the 'American Mosaic' of diverse cultures
reveals a healthcare arena of conflicting principles, values, and beliefs. For
many patients and practitioners, cultural worldviews not only exert a con-
spicuously powerful influence but also challenge assumptions we may have
regarding the universality of Western medical ethical principles such as individual patient autonomy. And because Others from non-mainstream cultures
may experience an increased risk of poor or ineffective healthcare service
due to misinterpretation, stereotyping, lack of understanding, and outright
discrimination, U.S. healthcare and regulatory measures now underscore the
importance of promoting cultural sensitivity and knowledge, or "cultural
competence" in an effort to bridge cultural fault lines between providers and
patients, and to close those gaps in awareness, understanding, and sensitivity.
These fault lines are not generated primarily by cultural differences them-

selves, but by difficulties in attitudes, skills, understanding, and communicating regarding differences. Consider Anne Fadiman's heart-wrenching account of Foua Yang, Nao Kao Lee, and their daughter Lia, Hmong refugees from the mountains of Laos who settle in California and encounter an alien health system with little understanding of their Hmong culture. Lia was three months old when she was diagnosed with epilepsy and treated with medications such as Valium and Depakene, much to the alarm of her parents who believed that Lia was experiencing *quag dab peg* ("the spirit catches you and you fall down"). They therefore sought to "fix her spirit" through traditional practices of animal sacrifice and rubbing coins on Lia's body. For several painful years, Lia's parents encountered a labyrinth of misunderstanding, during which time Lia suffered a massive seizure leading to her brain death.[1]

This points to a deeper, original fault line—the ever-widening chasm between our concerns and those of the Other, a fissure that intensifies as Western biomedicine continues to dominate the U.S. health system under the assumption of some common morality. Yet, as Leigh Turner points out, "Platitudes about common moral intuitions merely obscure the variable visions of moral life to be found in contemporary North America."[2] This book attempts to uncover and explore this deeper fault line.

This original fissure remains hidden from our vision primarily because we suffer from a socio-cultural anesthesia. We ignore, disregard, or disacknowledge what we somehow sense when it comes to those Others, who are habitually of less concern to us, that is until it comes to our own house, our hospital, our shores. As of this writing, there are ever-growing fears in the U.S. that unsafe levels of radiation from Japan's March 11, 2011, unprecedented and catastrophic earthquake-tsunami-nuclear calamity will soon be reaching our West Coast. Moreover, our attention is instinctively selective. Who and what we attend to reflects who and what matters to us. Inattention thereby always accompanies attentiveness. Yet our deliberate inattentiveness can also make us complicit in the Other's burden, so that we readily normalize the pathological and rationalize legitimacy purely on the grounds of common disposition and practice.

This is particularly the case with marginalized populations like the elderly. Through socially sanctioned labeling—"he's getting old," "it's all part of aging"—tagging each individual elderly patient as "old" first and "patient" second is the easier path. It takes an earnest effort to uncover the hidden and discover the particularity of this unique individual person who happens to be a patient who is elderly. Even though we intuit that not all elderly are "old," it requires a labor of forgetfulness to put this aside, especially in the volatile clinical setting where individualities, not categories, really matter.

It requires effort to *not* see the particular, unique Other who is before us in the clinical encounter. More literally, as I later explain, Emmanuel Levinas prompts us that the Other's face, or *visage*, embodies the Other's immediacy and presence to us. In this spirit of the patient's *visage*, the chapters' opening vignettes offer faces of patients, their families, and professional caregivers in tensions which embody chapters' themes. And each chapter charts a path to the text's overall course: as a necessary condition for cultural awareness, sensitivity, and competency in healthcare, we especially need to recognize and critically reflect on the complex problematic of the clinical encounter with the Other.

Our opening chapter reminds us of the blunt and oftentimes bitter reality of colliding worldviews. This clash of worldviews represents one of the most critical challenges we face in the arena of healthcare. This chapter presents the problematic surrounding the meaning of culture and discusses how the idea of culture is oftentimes poorly construed. In view of this and the tensions that can erupt among healthcare providers, patients, and their families, chapter 2 explores how, despite the need for some measure of "cultural competency," the notion itself suffers from lack of conceptual clarity and requires further unpacking. It goes on to examine morally compelling reasons for acquiring cultural competency within healthcare, and here we underscore the intrinsic link between culture and value in view of three critical dimensions of space, time, and modes of communication. Chapter 3 argues that cultural discourse, or conversation, is a necessary though in itself insufficient ground for cultural competence. It explores fundamental conceptual hurdles in cultural discourse, hurdles which affect clinical and institutional behavior and which we need to address in cultural competency work. Despite the benefits of cultural competency, one major peril lies in the issue of accommodation, or tolerance, of certain cultural behaviors that may be morally or institutionally intolerable. This chapter concludes by further examining tolerance and its limits.

In chapter 4, as a crucial component to address these hurdles I propose that we cultivate what I think of as the virtue of presence, an interpersonal, face-to-face engagement or being-with the patient. Levinas' metaphysics of the moral nature of personal engagement is especially relevant. The biggest challenge we face today in implementing presence lies in our socio-cultural default reliance on communication via technologies as a substitute for the interpersonal. In the final chapter, I highlight some rather basic and evident clinical strategies to help cultivate presence. As a start, I acknowledge that any attempt to foster interpersonal presence occurs within a prevailing climate of public distrust in our healthcare system. Nonetheless, we still yield to institutional and professional authority. After examining uncritical deference to this authority, I conclude with practical strategies, reaffirming that the quintessence of cultural competency lies in embracing, enhancing, and sustaining the humane quality of the healthcare provider-patient relationship.

These reflections come from my sustained and invaluable experience in healthcare settings with patients, their families, and their professional care-givers (physicians, nurses, social workers, psychiatrists, clergy, and ethics committees). As a philosopher by passion I remain unshakably confident in Epicurus' immortal admonition—"Vain is the discourse of that philosopher by whom no human suffering is healed." In our effort to reorient our field of vision to encompass the Other, when the Other's suffering fades away from recognition, we must out of necessity restore our sight and remind ourselves of what we cannot afford to neglect, otherwise we relinquish our humanity.

NOTES

1. Anne Fadiman, *The Spirit Catches You and You Fall Down* (New York: Farrar, Straus and Giroux, 1997).

2. Leigh Turner, "Zones of Consensus and Zones of Conflict: Questioning the 'Common Morality' Presumption in Bioethics," *Kennedy Institute of Ethics Journal*, 13, 3 (2003): 216.

Chapter One

When Worldviews Collide

Long ago in relative time, in September 2003, the new hit "reality" show, *Extreme Makeover*, entered its second season on ABC television. Millions of Americans watched as identical twins Caroline and Catherine, or "Cat," and 40 year-old Dan morphed into 'new' persons. Unhappy with her nose and smile among other things, Caroline underwent a chin implant, lower eyelid surgery, lowering of her upper lip, breast augmentation, liposuction of her thighs, tummy tuck, and dental work of gum re-contouring, root canals, and twelve porcelain veneers. Cat, annoyed at her post-pregnant tummy, subjected herself to liposuction of her thighs, breast augmentation, and a tummy tuck. Family and friends cheered and celebrated at the twins' "reveal party" afterwards. Single-dad Dan, displeased with his body and desperately wanting his office assistant to fall in love with him, stoically underwent Lasik surgery, hair transplantation, facial restructuring, a chin implant, and liposuction of the face, chest, belly, and love handles.

Aided by cosmetic surgeons, liposuctionists, cosmetic dentists, physical trainers, nutritionists, stylists, and fashion experts (they collectively called themselves the "Extreme Team"), the trio turned from drab and dowdy to attractive and alluring, at least in their eyes and in the eyes of millions of American viewers, or better, voyeurs. *Extreme Makeover*'s motto is blunt: "We'll stop at nothing to turn ordinary into extraordinary!" Here, our wildest dreams about how we desire to look can now come true—all things are possible. Progress without limits.

This transformation of the ordinary into the special embodies (no pun intended) the astonishing capacities and powers of our technologies of enhancement. The show's slogan hooks into the depths of our collective psyche, the unfulfilled desires and dreams of the mass of Americans who are made to feel as though they should not simply settle for the ordinary, the way they naturally look. The show's Disney-like message to viewers that fairy tales can come true helps explain *Extreme Makeover*'s phenomenal success, spawning spin-offs like *The Swan* and *I Want a Famous Face*, all the while fashioning the delusion that it is not personality and character that inspire self-confidence, success, affection, fame, and fortune. Instead, it is physical appearance.

Triumph, as always, has its price. Progress entails regress. *Extreme Makeover*'s extraordinary appeal, not just in our culture but in others, casts a sour indictment of an increasingly commonplace societal view, namely that how we feel about ourselves rests less upon how we *actually are*, but is determined more by *how we think others see us*. This calls to mind the murderer Garcin's poignant discovery in Jean-Paul Sartre's *Huis Clos* (*No Exit*). After villains Garcin, Inez, and Estelle, strangers to each other while alive, realize that they are now dead and condemned to remain forever with each other, thus constituting hell, Garcin declares:

> So this is hell. I'd never have believed it. You remember all we were told about the torture-chambers, the fire and brimstone, the "burning marl." Old wives' tales! There's no need for red-hot pokers. Hell is—other people! [1]

L'enfer c'est les autres. Recall the scene when Estelle awkwardly smudges her lipstick on her lips using Inez's eyes as a mirror. There are no mirrors in hell, no need for mirrors. We create our own hell when we define who we are on the basis of how we think others see us.

During that same week in September, millions throughout the world heard news reports of the impending execution of a thirty-one year-old Nigerian woman, Amina Lawal, who had given birth to her baby girl over a year after her divorce. She was arrested, tried, and found guilty of adultery by a local Shariah court on March 22, 2002. The Shariah court applied its own ruling in a rather harsh interpretation of Islamic law and sentenced her to death, death by stoning. Meanwhile, Yahay Mohammed, Amina's partner, though at first he admitted that he was the father of her child, later retracted his statement and denied paternity. He did not stand trial. His own personal oath was proof of his innocence.

Death by stoning is by all accounts gruesome, one of the most inhumane and degrading of executions. The intent behind stoning is to inflict as much pain as possible until the victim dies. The target is first buried up to her breasts. Stoners then hurl fist-sized rocks at her head, face, and upper body. These rocks need to be the right size, not too big and not too small. The Iranian penal code, for instance, is very specific about the size of stones to be used. With luck, the victim is quickly knocked unconscious. The stoning continues until the victim is dead. In many instances, the act is so brutal and prolonged that her head is nearly battered off.

When Amnesty International and other human rights and women's groups learned of Amina's plight along with that of other women awaiting a similar execution, they brought this to world attention. Amina's case was appealed, and on September 25, 2003, she was finally acquitted of the charges on legal technicalities. Nonetheless, to this day many others, mostly women, still await their execution by stoning.

These two accounts reveal a painfully stark contrast in worldviews. When *Extreme Makeover* announced its second season, thousands of Americans applied to be selected. Caroline, Cat, and Dan, among the chosen few, were awarded their new looks, their new faces, what many even consider their new identities. In another part of the world, Amina, singled out and imprisoned for her "dishonor," was in imminent danger of having her face ripped away. Others found guilty of similar crimes remain in jeopardy. For them, there is little concern for the wonders of cosmetic surgery, dentistry, Botox, skin peels, and laser treatments. The incongruity is all-too-raw.

WORLDVIEWS AND CULTURE

This opening chapter reminds us of what we already know—that worldviews can clash in significant ways. By worldview, I mean a conditioned and culti-vated perspective of reality as to what is most, more, and least important. A worldview entails considerations about what is valued, what matters. A worldview tackles questions like: What are the aims in life? What are the most significant means to achieve those aims? Who am I? Who are we? How are we to understand who we are? How are we to understand who we are in relation to others? How are we to live and behave with others? What does it mean to be good; what does it mean to be bad? All cultures offer their own unique responses to these questions so that each culture has its own world-view. To illustrate, our Western intellectual heritage underscoring a strict body-mind division has impacted the development of Western biomedicine in ways that biomedicine's ultimate goal lies essentially in ridding the body of pathologies, divorced from the wider context of the patient's embedded world of family, work, and relationships. Though this longstanding philo-sophical, religious, and scientific conviction affects the worldviews of U.S. health professionals, this body-mind separation is less evident among Asian traditions which acknowledge body-mind's mutually symbiotic link, and which in turn significantly affect Asian worldviews regarding illness and healing,

While worldviews shape metaphysical, ontological, and ethical perspec-tives, these domains are not siloed and compartmentalized from each other. Views of reality and views of identity naturally impact upon each other. How we view Being indelibly affects how we think of ourselves as beings within Being. Moreover, how we see ourselves will naturally bear upon how we believe we ought to live and act with others, those others who are like ourselves and those others who are not like ourselves, that is, the Other.

"Culture" can stand further unpacking. Clearly, while various cultures have their worldviews, and these worldviews are frequently at odds with each other, as within our healthcare settings, we need to exercise caution. If we define culture strictly along national, geographic, and religious boundaries, the relation between culture and worldview is asymmetrical since conflicting worldviews need not necessarily represent conflicting cultures. Colliding worldviews often occur within the same culture, as between Orthodox and Hasidic Jews within Jewish culture, or between Shiites and Sunnis within Islamic tradition. As defined above, cultures possess neither homogenous nor static values. In its broadest sense, culture signifies a dynamic situatedness-in-the-world so that there are distinct local worlds within, say, Japanese who live in Kyushu and those who live in Hokkaido. Local festivals, *matsuri*, are an expressive celebration of this unique situatedness. As Watsuji Tetsuro makes clear in his *Fudo*, climate, both meteorological and social, acts as a permanent marker on inhabitants' worldviews. Where we live affects how we live, what we live for, and what matters so that these local worlds represent subcultures, in lively tension with societal contexts that affect factors such as gender, age, status, power, and privilege. Herein lies the flow of culture, a dynamic, steady indeterminacy that resists fixed systems of values and beliefs. Arthur Kleinman reminds us of this:

> Culture, then, is built up out of the everyday routines and rhythms of social life. It is the medium of collective experience, for example, in which chronic pain affects an entire work unit, Alzheimer's disease is shared as an illness reality by a family, and pediatric cancer care is negotiated among parents, child, and professional care givers.[2]

To presume that culture constitutes an unchanging pattern of beliefs is a fatal flaw in cultural studies. To believe that a specific culture consists of a shopping list of traits is unashamedly simplistic. Culture does not comprise an unchanging bundle of values, beliefs, and practices. Thinking that it does plummets us into stereotypes, a mortal error in intercultural healthcare ethics. Hence, a foremost rule in intercultural studies: Culture does not represent an unchanging catalog of principles, values, beliefs, and behavior. A later chapter more closely examines this in light of certain hurdles to overcome in order to cross cultural fault lines and cultivate some measure of cultural competency.

Having said this, we can still claim distinct features of cultures in reasonably making generalizations, particularly since generalizations are a way of organizing our thoughts about culture and worldviews. Namely, we can plausibly assert that, first, cultures tend to embody certain worldviews, beliefs and values specific to those cultures, and furthermore, these worldviews often come into tension with each other in ways that lead to colliding values. Our two above vignettes share common ground in the brute fact of suffering. Caroline, Cat, and Dan suffer from poor self-esteem deriving in large part from what they think others think about their physical appearance. Amina suffers from an oppressive interpretation of the law that treats men and women inequitably. At the same time, the nature of their suffering and their responses to it differ, deeply colored by their respective cultural worldviews. The clash of worldviews is evident. Millions of Americans live vicariously through shows like *Extreme Makeover* and believe that enhancement technologies can make their dreams come true. Millions of Nigerian women no doubt dream of someday being free from the thumb of oppression. The clash between our culture's passionate consumerism and the Other's fundamental quest in eking out an existence is agonizingly palpable.

WORLDVIEWS AND HEALTHCARE

There is no dearth of dissonant worldviews in healthcare. Indeed, when it comes to healing, colliding worldviews constitute one of the most critical challenges we will continue to face throughout this century. To illustrate, consider these scenarios.

Rosa

When Rosa, a twenty-six-year-old Mexican mother, brought her two-month-old baby daughter to the emergency room at a Detroit hospital, the physician noted that the baby had high fever, dehydration, and sepsis. This explained why the baby had not been nursing and had regular bouts of diarrhea. The physician informed Rosa that her baby needed to have a spinal tap. He requested her signed consent. Rosa refused to sign the consent form, insisting that she could not do so without her husband's permission. This was the custom among Mexican households, particularly in important matters such as healthcare. In this case, her husband was out of town, and, for her baby daughter, time was of the essence.

Aksin

Aksin, a thirty-three year-old male Muslim from Turkey was admitted to a Kansas City hospital in order to undergo biopsies of suspicious tumors along his spine. Throughout his stay in a semiprivate room, the nursing staff found it extremely difficult to work with him. In their opinion, Aksin treated them condescendingly, constantly ordering them around, demanding their attention to even the most trivial details. In addition, even after visiting hours were over, family members still filled his room. And instead of following his prescribed medical diet, he often ate food given to him by his family. When it became clear that Aksin would not comply with their instructions, some nurses refused to work with him and informed their supervisor.

Rachel

As a Christian Scientist, Rachel, six-months pregnant, objects to surgical intervention and to any form of genetic tampering. Amniocentesis reveals that her fetus is abnormal with a rare metabolic disease due to a missing enzyme. Without intervention, Rachel's baby will most likely be born severely mentally disabled. Her physician recommends a new form of gene therapy which will introduce a gene into her fetus that will produce the needed enzyme. However, due to her strong religious beliefs, she refuses intervention, instead insisting upon the power of prayer and God's will.

Ly

Soon after Ly, a twenty-seven year-old Vietnamese man, was pronounced brain dead after being hit by a car while riding his bicycle, he was placed on life support until his family could be informed. His wife and parents soon arrived at the Los Angeles trauma center where an interpreter told them of his condition. They immediately left the center, and, because the staff neurosurgeon who would pronounce Ly officially dead was performing surgery, Ly remained on the ventilator. Shortly afterwards, the family returned and met with the interpreter and another physician. They had consulted an "expert," an astrologer (*bomoh*) who read Ly's astrological chart and strongly advised that his death be "postponed" until a more suitable time. According to Vietnamese beliefs, if a person died at the "proper" time, this would bring about good fortune and good health for that person's family. On the other hand, if a person died at the wrong time, this would spell misfortune for the family. According to the bomoh's interpretation of Ly's astrological chart, his death needed to be delayed.[3]

Jamila

Jamila, a thirty-eight year-old Egyptian Muslim female patient with Hodg-kins disease has been in a coma for the past three days as a result of anoxic encephalopathy, or severe loss of oxygen to her brain. The medical staff eventually approached the family to discuss the possibility of foregoing fur-ther life-saving treatment, treatment that they regarded as medically futile. The patient's family was horrified by the medical staff's conversation and request and was deeply suspicious of their motives. The family and Jamila were devote Muslims and had unreserved faith in the will of Allah. They perceived any consideration about withdrawing treatment as signaling aban-donment of Jamila. They refused to speak any further about the issue.

James

African Americans have good reason to be suspicious of U.S. government-run hospitals. The infamous Tuskegee trials where black males with syphilis were deliberately left untreated in the course of experiments helped to create a deep-seated legacy of distrust. So when James, a sixty-eight-year-old black male, had to undergo surgery for his prostate cancer, he suffered tremendous anxiety, refused to sign the hospital's consent form, and demanded to know more about alternative treatments. James had heard about the Tuskegee ex-periments and did not want to be another exploited human guinea pig.

Farmtha

Farmtha, a forty-two year-old Mien female, went to the local clinic with her fourteen year-old son as her interpreter. From her son's description of Farm-tha's symptoms—increased thirst, more frequent urination, tiredness—it ap-peared that his mother might be diabetic. A blood glucose test was in order, and a nurse soon approached the mother to draw her blood. At the sight of the needle, Farmtha screamed and refused to have her blood drawn. She and her son immediately left the clinic. Nurses shared this incident with a physi-cian of Mien descent. The physician told them that, according to Mien be-liefs, blood is associated with strength. Losing blood would mean losing strength. The mother was not frightened by the needle, but by the prospect of losing blood.[4]

* * *

When persons seek help for their health problems, they want to know two things: What is wrong? What can be done about it? They seek the opinion and advice of an expert healer. The expert's task is to address these two questions. The healer attempts to discover the problem, and, upon detecting the problem, he or she can then determine how it can be treated. Therein lies the healer's training, and the healer's art. And it is often the case that there is more than simply one way to treat the problem, more than one answer as to what can be done about it.

Knowing what *can* be done about it is one thing. Knowing what *should* be done, however, is another. What *ought to be done* is where moral conflicts come into play. Surely, what should be done will hinge very much upon the advice and counsel of the expert. Yet it will also rest upon what the patient and, in many cases, the patient's family determines—whether to go along with the healer's advice or to take another course. This is where values other than those of the expert enter in. The moral question regarding what *should* be done is not simply a matter of medical necessity, professional advice, and empirical evidence. Once other values, personal and cultural, enter into the picture, healthcare's terrain becomes more complex and challenging. Values about health, illness, well-being, and suitable treatment do not arise in a vacuum, but stem from the patient's worldview, his or her history, philosophical and religious beliefs, and social contours.

The above scenarios merely offer a glimpse into American healthcare's byzantine landscape of disparate assumptions and expectations about the nature of health, illness, etiology, the relationship between health and morality, family, gender roles, authority, age and the life-cycle, death, and grief. Not only does the patient population in the U.S., particularly in our metropolitan hospitals, come from numerous, diverse cultures, but the same is true for our healthcare professionals. This should come as no surprise in a U.S. population where more than 25% comprises African Americans, Asians, Latinos, and Native Americans. Unless we are prepared to acknowledge and come to terms with the fact of our American healthcare mosaic, we will not adequately address the healthcare needs of the communities we serve.

In this American mosaic, marginalized groups like the elderly, mentally and physically disabled, children, and minorities remain subject to unfair distribution of healthcare resources. With nearly 45 million Americans who remain uninsured, with most of them working uninsured, with an excess of inequity already within our healthcare system, can we attain a fair and just system of health? Whether or not a just health system is possible, it continues to be the case that in the absence of increased awareness, sensitivity, and responsibility to our marginalized groups, particularly those who come from non-mainstream cultures, our hospitals, clinics, psychiatric centers, long-term care facilities, and doctors' offices risk providing diminished and suboptimal healthcare. And this danger rests very much upon misinterpretation, lack of understanding, and stereotyping.

Any effort to bring about cultural sensitivity and responsiveness, what is termed "cultural competence," faces some rather daunting hurdles. For one, it is evident that we cannot realistically expect all healthcare professionals to know all there is to know health-wise about the beliefs, values, habits, and customs of their patient population. Not even scholars who have made it their career and lifeblood to examine various cultural beliefs and values can know all there is to know. Nevertheless, we need to start somewhere.

STARTING WITH OUR OWN HOUSE

Cultural competency begins with a two-fold recognition. First, we need to acknowledge that cultural competency is no final product. It is a life-long process, a never-ending journey with no end-point. Second, cultural competency starts with us. That is, we need to understand our *own* culture. Western biomedicine, with its set of beliefs and values, constitutes its own culture and worldview. Unless we can understand our own biomedical starting point, particularly here in the U.S., we can never genuinely engage in serious dialogue with the health-related beliefs and values of patients from other cultures. Cultural competency demands more than just cultural awareness and sensitivity. This being so, the first significant step toward cultural competence is to start with our own house.

The relationship between culture and healthcare is certainly evident in Western biomedicine, described as "one ethnomedicine among many others."[5] As such, certain prominent themes comprise the worldview of Western biomedicine, themes that oftentimes come into conflict with the worldviews of patients from other cultures.[6] Acknowledging these themes will contribute toward understanding the nature of the intercultural conflicts that we encounter in our healthcare.

One theme lies in Western biomedicine's tendency to *physicalize* illness and disease in that it aims to rid the patient of these via the patient's body. Causation is generally construed as organic, even in mental illness. Perhaps with the exception of family medicine, there is by and large little emphasis upon treating the person as a complete entity having bodily, spiritual, mental, and social moorings. Due to its overemphasis upon the physical, biomedicine disregards or minimizes other significant considerations. For the Mien mother who shows symptoms of diabetes, conducting the blood glucose test makes perfect medical sense. But if we attend to the fact that Farmtha is more than just her body, and that people from various cultures attach a special importance to certain aspects of their bodiliness, in this case blood, then the Mien mother's immediate revulsion also makes sense. In the same way, for the Vietnamese patient, Ly, and for his family, life is more than simply his body, so that the empirical determination of the permanent dysfunction of a bodily organ like the brain may indicate "death" in a clinical sense, but not necessarily in what others believe to be the real sense.

Biomedicine utilizes the language of organic affliction in determining that we are victims of our own bodily dysfunctions. In so doing it plays down social and cultural influences, including diet, lifestyle, environment, occupation, and religious belief. In fact, the more etiologies become shrouded in what is essentially uncertain and unknown, for example with cancer and depression, the more biomedicine reinforces a facile organic explanation. Given our prevailing conception of depression as a neurochemical disorder, and surely there is much to be said for the need for neurochemical balance in order to avoid the adverse effects of imbalance, biomedicine risks underestimating more profound questions as to sources for such imbalance. Now used even to treat minor distress, regular doses of Prozac only take us so far in treating depression.

As a second theme, biomedicine fundamentally *individualizes* by viewing all patients as independent, distinct, separate entities. This is consonant with Western culture's habit of privatizing each person, considering each person as a separate being. Because of this individualization, hospital staff naturally have difficulty comprehending Rosa's need to obtain her husband's permission before signing the consent form for her baby daughter. As in many Latino families, Mexican households tend to place less emphasis upon individual and private expressions of self-determination, or autonomy. Instead, when it comes to decision-making for family members, particularly in matters of health, the family plays the more important role with the father as the family spokesperson.

To further illustrate, Ruiping Fan cites the radical divergence between a Western liberalist individualism and the Confucian emphasis on family autonomy.[7] Fan's example is striking in view of our Western emphasis on individual patient self-determination and decision-making. Our emphasis upon appointing a single, specific individual family member as a surrogate decision-maker, a healthcare durable power-of-attorney, though sensible in our Western individualist context, within a Confucian context stands in danger of disrupting family cohesiveness as an interactive, interdependent, collective web. And what jeopardizes family harmony is antithetical to Confucian teaching. As Fan states:

> When the whole family makes medical decisions for the patient even when the patient is competent, it is only appropriate that the whole family continues to shoulder the obligation when the patient becomes incompetent. It would be woefully embarrassing for the Chinese to designate one family member, ignoring others, to be one's single decision maker. To do this is to destroy the unity and harmony of the entire family.[8]

Along these lines, to presume that certain Western bioethical principles lay the foundation for a global bioethics constitutes moral arrogance. In this brief study, I propose that a reasonable foundation for an intercultural discourse on healthcare ethics lies in our commonly shared embodied interpresence with, to, and for each other as a noncontingent interhuman biological and social reality and identity. Our inflated tendency to individualize also helps to explain our resistance to the Vietnamese family's reliance upon the advice of the *bomoh* and their demand that Ly be proclaimed dead at a more suitable time. Here there is more at stake than simply Ly's death, namely the fortune or misfortune of his family. Moreover, acquiring this sort of cultural understanding does not mean uncritically embracing specific customs, beliefs, and practices such as the burdensome patriarchalism in Latino cultures or the testimony of the *bomoh* in Vietnamese tradition. This naturally raises questions of tolerance and accommodation. How far can we justifiably go in our healthcare system in accommodating other cultures' values and beliefs? This remains one of the real plaguing concerns in efforts at cultural competency. We will reserve this issue of the limits of accommodation and tolerance for later discussion.

Third, biomedicine confers authority to biomedical *technology* in that it typically favors technological interventions over those that are more interpersonal. This is consistent with the broader cultural ethos among Americans who display a nearly blind faith in technology. This has been referred to as our "technological imperative," that is, the assumption that since we do have the technologies at our disposal, their only value lies in their application. This makes sense for our thoroughly pragmatic culture whereupon value is contingent upon usefulness. Medical technologies are no exception. In the case of Rachel, the well-being of her baby is at stake, and her physician and many on the medical staff are predictably puzzled by her refusal of the gene therapy that is available. At the same time, whether or not they consider her reliance upon God's will irrational, her situation especially warrants interpersonal intervention equally if not more so than technical. Sensitive and compassionate discussions with other family members and with the hospital chaplain would most likely help. Interpersonal rather than technological intervention also makes sense in James' case. The historical basis behind his skepticism regarding surgery for his prostate cancer provides further reason to discuss his options with him openly and honestly rather than immediately insisting that he undergo surgery.

Fourth, biomedicine is ultimately *crisis-oriented* in that it assigns a higher value to curing rather than to preventing illness and disease. This is the case despite the high potential for cost-containment through prevention. In the case of Jamila, the Egyptian in a coma, the medical staff initiated discussion about end-of-life decision-making once they determined that her treatment was medically futile. Within Western biomedicine, conditioned to think in terms of saving life and curing illness and disease, questions surrounding futile treatment present a special type of moral quandary for all the parties involved—patients, professionals, and families. Sadly, it is often the routine in most hospitals that medical staff will initiate this sort of discussion when things are at their worst for the patient. As long as conversation regarding end-of-life decision-making occurs when the situation is already clinically suboptimal, this will remain a plaguing issue. Resolving ethical conflict in healthcare cannot afford to simply take place ad hoc, but must also be preventive. Yet, rather than cultivate a climate that encourages early discussion about death and dying, we tend to address the crisis only as it happens. Talk of this nature *must* begin earlier. At the same time, as in the case of Jamila and her family, timing needs to be sensitive to religious convictions and how such conversation may be interpreted by patient and family. With each of these themes, biomedicine's culture clearly mirrors its broader culture. Biomedicine's crisis-orientation especially reflects a deeper American cultural ethos, one that dreads death and dying and militates against anything associated with death such as aging. This is plainly the case with our focus on acute care rather than care for chronic pain and illness. Acute illness presents itself as more curable, and biomedicine is ready to step in as the medical lifeguard, a *Baywatch* medicine lending itself to a *Baywatch* ethics, ready at a moment's notice to step in and rescue.

However, biomedicine constitutes one healing culture among others. Cultural anthropologist Richard Shweder describes biomedicine as one of a number of "causal ontologies" to explain suffering. He goes on to describe other causal ontologies that are moral, sociopolitical, interpersonal, and psychological:

> a moral ontology of transgression/sin/karma, or a sociopolitical ontology of oppression/injustice/loss, or an interpersonal ontology of envy/hatred/sorcery, or a psychological ontology of anger/desire/intrapsychic conflict and defense. [9]

It is supremely naïve to assume that the values and beliefs underlying Western biomedicine are shared by peoples and cultures throughout the world. Views of health, illness, disease, and especially stages of life, living, dying, and death carry their own unique cultural imprints.

Bestowing universal legitimacy to biomedicine's values and beliefs is both wrongheaded and dangerous. In our population that is culturally, ethnically, religiously, and sexually pluralistic, imposing a cultural template is unfair and arrogant. This is doubly dangerous in healthcare. First, because patients are inherently vulnerable, due to their discomfort, pain, and suffering, they need proper care and look to the healer for help. Second, on account of factors such as education, social status, and income, the healthcare setting is unambiguously filled with disproportion so that patients are naturally disempowered. Restoring a balance requires empowering them in ways that recognize and respect who they are as persons. A significant part of who they are as persons rests upon their own personal, familial, social, and deeply cultural contexts and narratives. Ignoring or discounting this injures them in ways that cannot be remedied through biomedical treatment. Cultural pluralism in our healthcare system is a major challenge that health professionals face. It is a challenge we all face and one we cannot afford to ignore.

NOTES

1. Jean-Paul Sartre, *No Exit and Three Other Plays* (New York: Random House, Vintage International, 1989), 45.

2. Arthur Kleinman, *Writing at the Margin: Discourse Between Anthropology and Medicine* (Berkeley: University of California Press, 1995), 54.

3. The cases of Rosa, Aksin, Rachel, and Ly are derived from Michael C. Brannigan & Judith A. Boss, *Healthcare Ethics in a Diverse Society* (Mountain View, CA: Mayfield Pub. Co., 2001), 171, 172, 247, 546.

4. The cases of James and Farmtha are based on Geri-Ann Galanti, *Caring for Patients from Different Cultures: Case Studies from American Hospitals*, 2nd ed. (Philadelphia: University of Pennsylvania Press, 1997), 5, 44.

5. R.A. Hahn, *Sickness and Healing: An Anthropological Perspective* (New Haven: Yale University Press, 1995),132.

6. See Hahn, *Sickness and Healing*, 142ff.

7. Ruiping Fan, "Bioethics: Communitization, or Localization?" in *Global Bioethics: The Collapse of Consensus*, ed. H. Tristram Englehardt, Jr. (Salem, MA: M & M Scrivener Press, 2006): 271–99.

8. Fan, 275.

9. Richard A. Shweder, *Thinking Through Cultures: Expeditions in Cultural Psychology* (Cambridge, MA: Harvard University Press, 1991), 315. Shweder cites the 1986 work of Arthur Kleinman, *Social Origins of Distress and Disease*, as a brilliant examination of how different cultures view suffering.

Chapter Two

From Fault Lines to Cultural Competency

Soon after his cataract surgery, Herminio, a fifty-five year-old Filipino patient, was restless, had difficulty sleeping, and showed the typical symptoms of discomfort and pain. Nurses offered pain medication, which he continued to refuse. He pointed out to them that they had other responsibilities, and he did not want to impose upon them. He also stated that everything is in God's hands, and that if God wishes for him to suffer pain, then it is God's will that he endure the pain. How should the nursing staff resolve this?

* * *

These colliding worldviews expose deep cultural fault lines that can erupt in strikingly perilous fashion. These fault lines are inevitable given the inseparable link between cultures and values and beliefs. Fault lines at times manifest irreconcilable worldviews with the potential to surface from a level of natural tension, as in the case of an African-American understandably distrusting a health system with its history of racial exploitation, to major conflict and apparent incompatibility, such as a Japanese family's adamant insistence on the use of a scarce resource, a ventilator, to keep their brain dead son 'alive.' These in turn reveal and give way to further social fractures, gaps that for Carolyn Nordstrom generate "flows" in inequity that "represent fissures in humanity."[1]

Nordstrom's analysis is instructive in emphasizing that fault lines, although distinct and culturally bound, also interact as the eruption of one affects others. Her extensive ethnographic research uncovers exploitative linkages intermingling marginalized groups' vulnerabilities and desperations, as in the extra-legal market in pharmaceuticals and medical supplies.[2] The same could be said for our worldwide use of cell phones, laptops, and other conveniences of information technologies. We obtain much of the needed mineral coltan through the labor of young children who mine coltan amidst internecine struggle in the Democratic Republic of Congo. Exploitation of marginalized groups is particularly evident when their vulnerability is both transformed and normalized through statistics that render marginalized humans as data, in effect invisible.[3] Indeed our original fault line, our Original Sin, lies ultimately in the chasm between our concerns and those of the Other, the Other referring to the unidentified, invisible behind the statistics, those over there, those whom we care not to care about, seemingly beyond our immediate moral concern, and, for many of us, outside of the moral community.

What Nordstrom calls "forging invisibility" thus constitutes a primordial fault line, a cheerless indictment of who we are, our propensity to look the other way regarding the suffering of Others, those outside of our own perceived moral community of concern. Stanley Cohen's incisive distinction between "knowledge" and "acknowledgment" is apropos.[4] *Knowing* that billions of persons are in need of basic and affordable healthcare to ward off preventable maladies like malnutrition and malaria entails a cognitive awareness from being informed. *Acknowledging* requires recognizing and incorporating that information, internalizing it in ways that compel us to act on what we know. As Cohen points out, we can rationalize away our knowing through "magical realism," convincing ourselves that what we know, for example, women being stoned to death for adultery, cannot really be happening since it falls outside the margin of what we consider legal and thus right, though morality and legality are discriminately distinct. Contorted reasoning of this sort situates victims outside the margin of the visible. It is one thing to know that people throughout the world starve to death in the tens of thousands each day, or will not have access to effective retroviral medicine in case of an H1N1 pandemic, or that countless African subjects of AIDS research can themselves never afford treatment once it is on the market. It is quite another to genuinely recognize these truths in ways that shake us from our zones of comfort. We see models for recognition and hope in the steady struggle and efforts of groups like *Medicins san frontiers* or individuals like Paul Farmer in Haiti. Nonetheless, and ironically in the case of child labor to mine coltan for our cell phones, we can use our ubiquitous connective technologies intended for us to more globally connect, to create and nourish our comfort zones. We essentially deny what we know and do not see that which is before us.

Consider Nordstrom's account of human trafficking with fault lines and linkages that are built-in so that we choose to not recognize them through various strategies that manufacture invisibility:

Visualize moving one gun, or girl, from birthplace to a site of labor. This requires a cast of hundreds: factory workers or "employment agencies" to "create a product"; people in bus, train, and shipping industries to move them, as well as agents at borders and ports; managers along the way to buy, sell, package—and in the case of the girl—feed, clothe, and tend; people to rent and sell houses and offices; others to maintain and repair commodities and provide medical treatment for the trafficked girl; companies that advertise and provide protection and enforcement; bankers and accountants to manage and launder profits; and, finally, lawyers to provide legal counsel. And the customers.[5]

Her account unveils the systemic character that accompanies "forging invisibility," and these systemic roles comprise a further fault line. The tattered fabric of our U.S. healthcare system, with its high percentage of uninsured and underinsured and a tiered system favoring the rich and affluent, combined with a biomedical ethos that essentially physicalizes illness and disease (maintaining a body-mind duality), individualizes patients as independent and separate entities, confers excess authority to technological interventions rather than interpersonal, and assigns higher value to curing rather than to preventing illness and disease, naturally lends itself to deep fissures.

Conventional wisdom all too easily places blame for such systemic fault lines upon party politics, lobbying groups, corrupt government, regimes, or foreign despots. Yet conventional wisdom is generally short-sighted, and stunted vision merely reinforces non-acknowledgment and characterizes the Serpent syndrome as in the Genesis account, blaming the serpent for biting the apple, our natural tendency (another original sin) to blame an external entity, an "it" or Other rather than looking for some measure of accountability within. Moral accountability is non-negotiable. Our humaneness demands it. The ripple effects of our confined commitment to only the here, now, and visible and not to what is "over there," about to come in the near and distant future, and what is invisible are undeniable. As in Plato's Cave, there are at least two ways we choose to know and see: first, via what we desire to see, and second through what we cannot help but see. Yet desires drive vision, and as David Hume incisively reminds us, this triumph of desires becomes customary through force of habit.

For these reasons, fault lines normally lie hidden. On the surface, we maintain a day to day pretense of normalcy, that is, until fissures eventually erupt. So how do eruptions occur? More importantly, why do they continue to occur? Cultural fault lines represent certain beliefs and values that not only affect ways we view healthcare, illness, death, morbidity, disease, aging, and health, but spawn fissures within our healthcare system, driven by its own ethos and worldview. And here is the rub. Eruptions within institutional and clinical frameworks often appear ethical in nature, lending themselves to the common parlance of "ethical dilemma." Yet how we frame the problem is a crucial part of our moral inquiry and understanding. All too often we frame an issue in language and terms of some sort of "ethical dilemma," as if there are essentially two no-win alternatives. This *dilemma mindset* is skewed, reductionist, ignorant of broader contextual issues, and simply wrong-headed. As many of us who have deliberated on hospital ethics committees know, eruptions often represent conflicts that are communicative—matters of nondisclosure, misunderstanding, absence of clarification, lack of follow-through, disconnect among various specialists, personal tiffs among health professionals, family turf battles, and so on. Surely, matters ethical and communicative, though distinct, are not separate. Communication and ethics are deeply interwoven in a relationship that up to now has not gleaned the attention and analysis it requires. On a more positive refrain, we are now seeing increasing institutional and collaborative efforts to explore the links between communication and ethics in healthcare such as Cardiff University's Health Communication Research Centre in Wales and the Indiana Center for Intercultural Communication at IUPUI (Indiana University–Purdue University Indianapolis.[6]

UNPACKING CULTURAL COMPETENCY

"Culture"

With cultural fault lines that increasingly surface among healthcare providers, patients, and their families, institutional necessity in the form of regulatory requirements involve establishing so-called cultural competency training for health professionals. Moreover, aside from the pragmatic aim of reducing medical liability, there are morally compelling reasons for fostering cultural awareness and sensitivity within healthcare, particularly the need to redress healthcare treatment inequities and unfair health outcomes due to cultural myopia and misunderstanding. However, though common parlance, the term itself suffers from an insufficient conceptually sound basis as to what constitutes a "culturally competent" healthcare professional. Definitions of cultural competency are often sketchy at best. The following characterization by Wen-Shing Tseng and Jon Streltzer in their helpful *Cultural Competence in Health Care* is typical.

> To provide cultural competent healthcare, providers need to have a culturally sensitive attitude, appropriate cultural knowledge, and flexible enough skills to provide culturally relevant and effective care for patients of diverse backgrounds.[7]

While this description properly subordinates the acquisition of knowledge and underscores the priority of attitude, it is still sparse and says little by way of generic terms. As a start, the notion of "culture" needs further unpacking. To elaborate upon remarks in the opening chapter, there are clearly various ways to construe "culture." In the most fundamental sense, human culture is a product of human design, a human construct distinct from the natural realm. Ernst Cassirer, through his marvelous metaphysics of the human as symbolic, stresses that humans simultaneously create culture through symbol—language, art, myth, religion, science—and understand themselves through these cultural creations and symbols. The human creates and refashions culture, and vice versa. Therein lies our human community. Within this human construct we may then view culture as patterns of values, beliefs, behaviors, and worldviews among humans. Matters of cultural competency refer precisely to this generic description of culture as a pattern of worldviews, beliefs, values, and dispositions that distinguish holders of these worldviews from holders of other worldviews. Culture is a segregative term demarcating one group from other groups, the effects of which naturally unfold, often in non-deliberative, unintended ways in perspectives concerning what comprises health, illness, healing, and death.

In this generic, segregative formulation, culture is distinct from 'race,' which is in itself a social construct, not indicative of biological and physiological differences as previously thought. Rather than 'race,' culture involves ethnicities, groups sharing a history and behavior patterns that form a distinct identity and that plays out in disproportional health dispositions, for instance when African-Americans tend to be more prone to sickle-cell anemia, Asians to stomach cancer, and Ashkenazi Jews to Gaucher's disease and Tay-Sachs. Within this segregative notion, Emmanuel Levinas speaks of cultures as fundamental "pathways" to meaning:

> All things picturesque in history, all the different cultures, are no longer obstacles that separate us from the essential and the Intelligible; they are the paths by which we can reach it. Furthermore, they are unique pathways, the only possible paths, irreplaceable, and consequently implicated in the intelligible itself![8]

Culture represents for us, whether within a culture or peering in from the outside, our avenue to understanding.[9] Furthermore, this generic and segregative view of culture admits of an inherent, unfolding dynamism so that culture is never static. Culture cannot be reified, transformed into a static, thing-like entity which occurs when we erroneously associate culture with a similarly reified sense of tradition.[10]

With this broad understanding of culture as a backdrop, the notion of cultural competency thus carries a particularly normative quality since culture in this generic sense assumes an interweaving of culture and value, expressed through three fundamental and interactive dimensions of space, time, and modes of communication. With respect to the dimension of space, spatiality provides the natural physical arena for interconnections and relations as evident in matters of family hierarchy, authority, and dynamics. In many cultures, such as Mediterranean and Islamic, family plays a leading role in providing care during illness. And African Americans tend to comprise a more matriarchal system with mother and/or grandmother as head of the family. Of particular spatial importance are the prominent distinctions among those who occupy various circles of intimacy and importance, as evidenced in the Japanese tradition in which there is a near sacrosanct line between insider, *uchi*, and outsider, *soto*. Furthermore, within the domain of spatiality, meanings attached to our physical body play a key role. As embodied beings, we live in and through our bodiliness, intrinsic to spaces within which we live. Views of bodiliness affect views of self and personal identity through perennial questions such as What is my self? What is the relationship between my body and self? What is the relationship between my body and my personal identity?

The dimension of time offers further context for considering human interaction in the light of values and beliefs. In the U.S., usefulness and productivity are leading values in view of our decidedly pragmatic orientation so that present and future tenses assume high importance. In our future-oriented society, we inheritors of the bold ambition of our early pioneers who sacrificed safety and comfort for future security aim to build a better future to achieve success. Our history underscores America as the land of promise. Therefore in the U.S., the death of an infant or of a young adult is thereby considered ultimately tragic. In a future-oriented society, early death represents the loss of the future, the death of promise, of potential. Here, of course, we need to be wary of overgeneralizing. Subcultures thrive within major cultural groupings. Hispanics and Asians tend to value traditions of the past. So also, Chinese culture with its rich and ancient history places great emphasis upon past and living tradition. This helps explain why Chinese view the elderly, whose living presence embodies a storehouse of past, tradition, and wisdom, with utmost respect, a striking expression of the Confucian teaching of filial piety. While in the U.S. the death of an elderly person is no doubt sad but nonetheless anticipated (though no matter how prepared we think we are, death still catches us off guard), for Chinese the death of an elderly person evokes heightened sorrow as it also represents the death of history, tradition, and sacred memory.

How we view time profoundly affects meanings we assign to life's natural stages so that different cultures view aging differently. Temporality shapes notions of family since values we place on extended family reflect degrees to which we value family lineage and history. Temporality clearly conjoins with spatiality as notions of family affect living arrangements, family dynamics, and family authorities, whether matriarchal or patriarchal.

As culture's third dimension, communication incorporates both spatiality and temporality. In writing a book on "How to Talk with Americans" what set of assumptions regarding space, time, and identity would it include?[11] Communication's complex matrix of verbal skills (dialects, volume, intonations) and nonverbal skills (body language, eye contact, distance, touch, particularly bodily contact between sexes, degrees of formality or familiarity, and gender), naturally involve spatial and temporal considerations. For instance, given the importance across cultures of protecting our own personal space, what does that personal space consist of? Formal greetings have a way of reflecting meanings we attach to this space, from making physical contact through shaking hands to refraining from such contact via bowing. So does eye contact.[12] In this communicative dimension, note differences in how persons from various cultures respond to and communicate pain. American Indians like the Navajo tend to treat pain stoically as a necessary part of life, in contrast to Italian Americans who are inclined to be more expressive.

"Competency"

Upon further inspecting the idea of culture, appreciating its intricacy and steering clear of reductionist simplification, we now face the question of competency. If healthcare professionals are called upon to exercise cultural competency, what does this entail? At first, this strongly suggests a sufficient knowledge base with respect to culture, ethnicity, race, religion, gender, issues regarding pain avoidance and expression, medication preferences (injections or pills), organ transplantation, and so on, one that can be practically applied in healthcare settings, including long-term care, with patients from various cultures. Acquiring this knowledge base is certainly helpful, for instance, when treating Muslim patients. For many Muslim patients, sensitivity to gender is especially critical. With strict requirements of segregation such as the expectation that female physicians alone should treat women, knowing relevant aspects of Muslim medical culture are crucial. Consider informed consent. Mainstream Western views of informed consent rest upon notions of self-determination, the meaning behind which often flounders when applied to Muslims. A physician's honest disclosure of the seriousness of a diagnosis may be viewed not only as unnecessary but harmful in diminishing the Muslim patient's level of hope, increasing patient apprehension, and conveying a sense of physician incompetence, as a result displacing trust in the physician's authority. Negative medical outcomes are generally viewed as the will of Allah so that end-of-life decision-making is especially difficult, particularly when physicians are expected to inform not the Muslim patient but the head of the family, who then decides any further course of action.

Yet, as alluded to earlier, acquiring a cognitive base of cultural views regarding health, illness, and so on, should not occupy top rank in a hierarchy of importance. Thinking that it does detracts from attending to the interpersonal dynamics in a face-to-face encounter with a patient which in turn requires proper attitude, the 'right stuff,' as a necessary first step. It is important to understand why many African-Americans' views toward a white, Caucasian dominated health system tend to be less trusting and more suspicious, given their history of exploitation, for example in the Tuskegee experiments, and in exclusion of African Americans from taking part in promising clinical drug trials and diets. Understanding this background may help to establish and cultivate rapport and trust. Yet knowing this past history of manipulation in itself does not bring about competency. More importantly, competency requires demonstrating a respectful attitude and applying interpersonal and communicative skills that can make the day, particularly in view of the ever-present reality of social and economic disparities among vulnerable groups of minorities, disabled, children, elderly, and other disenfranchised populations. This respectful attitude demands professional humility and self-questioning as to our own biases and cultural dispositions we bring to the bedside. Tseng and Streltzer remind us that "Physicians, nurses, social workers, and other healthcare providers need to be aware of their own cultural beliefs and biases to be cognizant of their own cultural sensitivity, and to examine the cultural relevance of the healthcare service they provide."[13]

To illustrate this cultural bias, not in order to judge right or wrong, consider our public consensus regarding brain death and organ transplants, of course aside from exceptions. The two are indelibly linked through identifying a brain death formula with what is considered clinical death, philosophical-religious scrutiny aside. Reaching this associative blueprint in the U.S. is historically sparked by organ transplant technologies' remarkable successes, advances in immuno-suppressive agents (from cyclosporine to FK506), and increasing emphases upon patient autonomy and individual choice to allow for one's own determination in end-of-life matters, particularly regarding the use and disposal of organs. As Margaret Lock deftly notes in her *Twice Dead: Organ Transplants and the Reinvention of Death*, cultural factors are clearly at play.[14] When compared and contrasted with the Japanese experience, what is intriguing is how readily acceptable and more routinized brain death and organ transplants have become in the U.S. where, following the first successful heart transplant in 1967 and more in its wake, as well as the passing of the Uniform Determination of Death Act in 1981, there was little, if any, public debate regarding either brain death or organ transplants (with the exception of some philosophical, theological pieces that did not gain ground in public discussion). Lock further points out that this routinization is particularly evident in the normalizing discourse using the "gift of life" metaphor, distinct from Japan's more evident and longstanding societal angst regarding bodily integrity, views of death, and heart transplantation.

This problematic regarding consensus is underscored by H. Tristram Englehardt in his instructive compilation, *Global Bioethics: The Collapse of Consensus*, where he rules out the possibility for crafting a global bioethics that can be universally applied to all cultures.[15] His analysis is thoughtful and persuasive and merits further comment, particularly since he also challenges any sound basis for a global morality. He stresses that the problematic of fault lines constituting "incompatible moral lifestyles embedded in disparate moral life-worlds" is fundamentally irresolvable on account of differing moral, metaphysical, epistemological, and logical premises. I offer an example. Arguing for a particular position regarding physician-assisted-suicide (or, more euphemistically, physician-aid-in-dying) entails a point of reference with certain premises regarding "harm," "patients' rights," "physician obligations," "nonmaleficence," and so on, that, wrapped in the reasoning for such position, according to Englehardt, *de facto* begs the questions as to the universal validity of these premises.

Despite this moral incommensurability, not to be associated with moral relativism, a prevailing rhetoric of "moral consensus" sustains the illusion of universal moral accord, a rhetoric which reflects a "studied pretense" that disparities and their underlying fault lines are superficial whereby real universal moral common ground exists. Englehardt illustrates this rhetoric of consensus by targeting the United Nations Educational, Scientific, and Cultural Organization's (UNESCO) 2005 Declaration on Bioethics and Human Rights, and cites Article 12:

> The importance of cultural diversity and pluralism should be given due regard. However, such considerations are not to be invoked to infringe upon human dignity, human rights and fundamental freedoms, nor upon the principles set out in this Declaration, nor to limit their scope.[16]

His critique of UNESCO's ungrounded presumption of consensus over the meanings of "human dignity," "rights," and "freedoms" parallels the critique that can be leveled against assumptions as to the universality of the so-called four principles of biomedical ethics (see appendix). It also parallels my overall critique of features of biomedicine.

As I see it, this pretense regarding moral consensus further legitimizes a moral imperialism, an inevitable side-effect of the cultural imperialism that is evident when Western cultural ideals (regarding beauty, fashion, progress, and so on) are exported without question and more subtly imposed on other cultures. This captures the insidious quality of globalization's liquefying effect upon culture, as Zygmunt Bauman puts it in his *Culture in a Liquid Modern World*, eroding their bases for solidity, stability, and security. [17] Due to the influence of post-modernism, what Bauman calls "liquid"modernity is a more appropriate designation as the image aptly captures our contemporary quandary—that is inventing our own anchor of stability in a world defined by flux and instability. This is the case especially in a Western biomedicine-bioethics nearly entirely secularized, lacking both *telos* and ultimacy. In this light, along with the rhetoric of consensus, the rhetoric of consumerism serves a marketing agenda and side-steps any impassioned discussion and disagreement that would naturally occur in public forums that sufficiently reflect diversity.

To further illustrate this rhetoric of moral consensus, Englehardt alludes to the plethora of ethics commissions/courses that seem to somehow reach consensus through rational discussion, discourse, and deliberation. He points out how implicit political and institutional agendae in effect establish com-mittees as a stacked deck providing the illusion of consensus. In my exten-sive and involved experience with hospital ethics committees as their desig-nated "ethicist," I've noted a prevailing committee dynamic in which "group think" is often the rule of order. Underlying tensions, often more subtle, including personality clashes, communicative breakdowns, authority road-blocks, systemic constraints, and professional caste power-plays tend to be covered up. Certain voices carry imbalanced authority, particularly those representing compliance, legal counsel (hospital counsel ought not to sit on such committees), and "ethics" from the "ethicist," all contributing to a cer-tain disingenuousness behind committee "deliberation." Under the veneer of consensus exist tensions regarding the smaller internal playing fields, and this is particularly the case with respect to matters of cultural competency. Efforts at consensus usually assume some privileged starting point with un-examined premises, from a basis in itself less exposed to critical self-exam-ination. For these reasons, we need more in-depth analyses regarding the natural relationship between communication and the complexities of dis-course and ethics.

In contrast to this cultural hubris and professional inability and unwilling-ness to be self-critical, a professional and "cultural humility" demands that we be especially aware of cultural biases that have long conditioned how we view moral issues and moral reasoning in ways that assume application of some rigid universal principles. [18] Hence the paradox in our assuming a moral framework that is itself culturally and historically derived. We can apply this to the relatively new interdisciplinary field of bioethics, itself the offspring of what was once medical ethics and later morphed into biomedical ethics.

Bioethics' interdisciplinarity is both its strength and its Achilles' heel. Unfortunately, in the U.S., as a field it appears to demonstrate less philosophical self-critique. One of its scholars Henk ten Have asserts:

> The fundamental ethos of applied bioethics, its analytical framework, methodology, and language, its concerns and emphases, and its very institutionalization have been shaped by beliefs, values, and modes of thinking grounded in specific social and cultural traditions. . . . Scholars usually assume that its principles, theories, and moral views are transcultural. [19]

Emmanuel Levinas warns against this conceptual hubris when he asks why Western philosophy exhibits this need to "absorb all Other in the Same, and neutralize otherness," a fundamental philosophical flaw that equally applies to bioethics. [20] Such leveling out or "neutralizing" of cultures reflects bioethics' inwardness, self-directed rather than other-directed. In view of the ever-present danger of stereotyping cultures and reifying culture as some "thing" for us to own in our understanding of cultural competency, we must not lose sight of the truth that we know ourselves upon going outward as long as there is a return to the self for self-critical assessment. This is the emphasis in cultural humility, rather than some more inflated notion of cultural competency. Simply put, reducing cultural competence to simply acquiring a knowledge base remains flawed. Particularly in cultural competency work, applying cognitive literacy rests upon proper attitude and appropriate skills. In this respect, what we will later examine more closely as the "virtue of presence" should permeate the clinical encounter. Otherwise, cultural competency efforts themselves become formulaic, superficial in the resolutely human encounter between the vulnerable patient and the officially empowered health professional, an encounter where lack of authenticity is likely to be detected by vulnerable patients. In order of importance, we can apply the triad of attitude-skills-knowledge, as in ASK, in which right attitude and sound communicative skills remain more important than acquiring a knowledge base. [21]

WHY CULTURAL COMPETENCY?

All of the above means that cultural competency in effect pertains to all patients, not just those from other cultures. Again, framing any issue is crucial for it sets the tone for how we think about it. If we frame cultural competency within a context of understanding and being more sensitive to those Others, in cultures outside of our own immediate locale, outside of our own private moral commune, the framing misleads. Surely, the need for understanding and sensitivity is excruciatingly vital in order to serve vulnerable populations and groups, like the elderly, mentally and physically disabled, minorities, immigrants, groups that are especially marginalized in mainstream Western biomedicine. As a whole, they suffer from diminished access to healthcare, lack of health insurance, disparate health outcomes due to insufficient attention, care, and increasing chronic and acute afflictions. For the marginalized, especially those trapped in the interlocked web of social poverty, oppression, limited healthcare access, and discrimination, each day represents a struggle to avoid any real health risk, a potential visit to an Emergency Unit, "just making it through the day." Cultural competency work out of necessity addresses the deep-rooted socioeconomic and systemic fault lines leading to health disparities.

Acquiring levels of cultural competence naturally entail somehow addressing health disparities in access and outcomes that come about because of cultural and ethnic insensitivity accompanied by lethal stereotyping and racial discrimination, all attributable to factors that include our own unquestioned biases, inability to communicate, ignorance, lack of knowledge, and negative attitudes.[22] Antonella Surbone says it well when describing cultural competency within the context of cancer care among cultures as grounded "on knowledge of the notion of culture; on awareness of possible biases and prejudices related to stereotyping, racism, classism, sexism; on nurturing appreciation for differences in healthcare values; and on fostering the attitudes of humility, empathy, curiosity, respect, sensitivity and awareness."[23] Furthermore, these attitudes operate within a systemic climate that funnels out in ways that impact individuals within the organization, so that cultural awareness is also a matter of organizational ethics.[24]

On account of accreditation requirements, cultural competency training occurs in residency programs and medical school curricula. Yet despite the plethora of training programs, attention to acquiring bodies of knowledge can swing attention away from what is more crucial, matters of attitude and skills. It bears repeating that cultural competency is more about attitude and communicative skill and sensitivity than acquiring a catalog of information. This has been evident for some time in transcultural nursing, a field of interest developed in the U.S. and in many ways a precursor to current cultural competency emphases.[25] Evidently nurses play various roles in different cultures. For example, the subordinate role of nurses in Thailand contrasts with the more active role for nurses in the U.S., especially since American nurses, in contrast to Thai nurses, have a collective support system that permits them to convey a more critical view of physicians' actions and decisions.[26]

Nurses play key roles in the front lines of patient care and interacting with family, and transcultural nursing studies remind us of the vital distinction between disease and illness. Without any doubt, Arthur Kleinman particularly stands out for his groundbreaking work on this.[27] Disease comprises a medical determination about illness with 'objective' parameters such as organic etiology and biological and physiological factors. Furthermore, there is an assumption of universality with respect to diseases. Epilepsy can be universally recognized, though not described as such. Illness, on the other hand, constitutes a patient's perception and experience of dysfunction and suffering. Here, things get sticky since the subjectivity of perception and experience does not lend itself to universal application, though cultural imprint plays a major role. Epilepsy, though a diagnostic category, is called by other names, as in seizures in the context of voodoo medicine or karmic effect in a Hindu worldview. Western biomedicine, institutionalized in mainstream U.S. healthcare, tends to view both disease and illness differently from more traditional approaches to healing, such as traditional Chinese medicine with its emphases on yin/yang harmony and *ch'i* balance, Indian Ayurvedic medicine, and Galenic Islamic emphases between healing and religious belief. As for this deep-rooted Islamic link between healing and religious expression, Muslims in particular tend to view healing as an important step in enabling the practice of the Five Pillars of Islam which also incorporate both familial and social roles. That is, salvation is never simply a personal matter, but entails obligations to the community, particularly to those who are more vulnerable and oppressed. Moreover, surrendering to Allah's will plays a major role for Muslim patients. In contrast to Western bioethics' emphasis on prior discussions regarding patients' will as in advance directives, such considerations may be viewed as antithetical to reliance on the will of Allah and deference to the authority of the physician.[28]

On account of its intercultural, transcultural, and universal focus, cultural competency requires a point of reference that transcends the local in an attempt to be global. If our point of reference remains confined to the parochial, our perspectives ignore healthcare's tangled web. We see the impact of globalization, for example, in the form of transnational interests invested in pharmaceutical companies. Cultural competency cannot help but consider healthcare within a global vision while at the same time recognizing that the entire range of global health is beyond our reach since it burrows into the full spectrum of economic, social, environmental, and political angles. Yet maintaining a global reference point in the best way we can uncovers an enormously complex labyrinth, providing all the more reason to challenge a simplistic and naïve notion of cultural competency as fundamentally equivalent to acquiring a knowledge base of cultures.

Sidestepping a global reference point, however, also permits us to normalize inequities so that we are complicit in manufacturing their invisibility. Unfortunately, it is only when fault lines erupt that we seek to disable what has been normalized. Even then, we may still think of it as "someone else's problem." We call in a cavalry of 'fixers,'—the interpreter, the "ethicist" (a now distorted and much abused term, the utterance of which has subtly morphed from describing to declaring), and clergy. For instance, the question "What is an 'ethicist'" naturally precedes the question "What does it mean to be a 'bioethicist?'"[29] If a certified "ethicist" or "bioethicist" is one who has successfully passed training hurdles, the certification itself does not warrant real life professional and practical competence.

Whether an intensive course of one or two weeks, or even a month, sufficiently prepares one to assume a leading voice in healthcare ethics is problematic.[30] Furthermore, upon considering the training process, dangers in reductionism, for example, via simplistic PowerPoint presentations, are increasingly evident. Whereas moral reasoning is inherently complex and nuanced, complex notions reduced to bullet points easily lead to bullet-point thinking[31] Certifying ethicists and bioethicists who will become prominent voices on hospital ethics committees and will engage in life and death ethics consults where the stakes are high is no small matter. As we read in Renée Fox and Judith Swazey's insightful sociocultural account, *Observing Bioethics*, bioethics has become a major cottage industry.[32] When conducted along these lines, the burgeoning business of ethics threatens to merely kayak over intricate and deep moral waters, skimming the surface of typologies, language, theories, and superficial application.

Note that this urge for someone else to "fix" the "problem" carries tentative and skewed assumptions regarding both the fixer and the problem. The interpreter acts as a cultural broker, the ethicist as ethics guide, and clergy as spiritual bridge (presuming a false dichotomy between secular and spiritual). In the spirit of Western biomedicine, we tend to address the rupture symptomatically without tackling the difficult task of digging into deeper causes. If ill-prepared with respect to the rupture (the problem), we are ill-equipped to address causes. The "problem," by the way, lies not with medical technologies. We cannot afford to undermine, minimize, or deride the powerful benefit of modern technological medicine. As Paul Farmer testifies regarding the medical marvel of heart surgery in Rwanda, "It was awesome medically . . . awesome personally . . . and it was awesome spiritually to see, on the exact anniversary of the 1994 genocide, that the power to heal continues to trump the power to maim, sicken, or kill."[33] The trouble lies not with our medical devices, but with how our relationship to our medical tools influences how we view ourselves, others, and how we relate to others.

At its heart, cultural competency signifies an epistemological and moral imperative to go beyond appearances and dig beneath the surface. Digging deeper discovers fault lines that underlie behaviors, institutions, and systems and have to do with profoundly personal and collective philosophical and religious beliefs and worldviews. As a case in point, meanings we assign to death reveal how, as Lock puts it, "margins between life and death are socially and culturally constructed, mobile, multiple, and open to dispute and reformulation."[34] Apologists for *Nihonjinron* (the genre stressing Japanese uniqueness and exceptionalism) often underscore their culture's distinctive perceptions regarding death: death not as individual and private but as social and relational, particularly familial; death not strictly in terms of the demise of cognition, consciousness, and awareness, but more in terms of biological constructs and the death of the body. Brain death may signify the irreversible loss of consciousness. But why would this matter in any significant way? Why focus on consciousness? As long as biological life persists, there remains life. The body is still 'living.'[35] In addition, meanings of death not only reflect meanings of life but influence and are influenced by views of individual identity in relation to others. Lived personhood is not exclusively individual but relational. The death of the person is also a relational, familial, and societal affair, a social occasion, not a medical determination of a moment in time. This helps to explain the prominent role of the family in Japan in deciding what to do with *itai*, the deceased's body, viewed relationally as a candidate for ancestry, not merely as *shitai*, a corpse, a thing.

Ripple effects of this bodily ontology reach into issues such as organ transplantation, considered in the U.S. as the ultimate "gift of life." In the U.S., from senseless tragedy (whether from natural causes, accidents, suicide, or homicide—the NASH formula for our death certificates), an intense personal, life-sustaining meaningfulness comes about through transplantation. Yet "gift" does not carry identical meanings across cultures, as seen in the value placed on the relationship between gift-giving and reciprocity, and, in Japan, reciprocity is expected to be of equal exchange value (why keeping labels on gifts continues to be important in Japanese gift-giving practice). Giving anonymously appears in itself to be rather odd so that within this perspective, what others elsewhere call the "gift of life" may be naturally viewed with suspicion. Even this high act of altruism may contain a hint of self-interest in the belief that the donor somehow 'lives' on in the recipient. All this naturally has profound existential and ontological significance. Our altruism, while virtuous within our Judaeo-Christian heritage, makes less sense to the Other.

In our quest of cultural competency, hidden epistemic issues concerning the fact/value distinction surface. Despite a strict medical determination of brain death, we cannot so easily divorce cold objectivity from the warm subjective realm of values. In matters medical, what qualifies as "evidence" rests upon socio-cultural assumptions regarding validity and truth. It also rests upon competing intellectual frameworks, embedded and constitutive of varying disciplines each with their own singular "styles of reasoning" (Ian Hacking's term). Can we culturally acknowledge the ambiguity of bodiliness, as in a body deemed "brain dead"? While globalization increasingly appears to represent a newly fashioned capitalist wedge designed to promote cultural singularity, varying reasoning styles remain. These "styles of reasoning" reflect ways we order the world, ways in which we make sense of ostensible nonsense, when we transform a tragic accident into a means to provide the "gift of life" to another. Thus the pure separation of fact and value is misconceived.[36] This fact/value relation is certainly apropos in medicine, a science that deals specifically with pain, suffering, health, and healing, and for this reason perhaps the most humane of the sciences.

NOTES

1. Carolyn Nordstrom, "Fault Lines," in *Global Health in Times of Violence*, ed. Barbara Rylko-Bauer, Linda Whiteford, and Paul Farmer (Santa Fe, NM: School for Advanced Research Press, 2009), 64.

2. Nordstrom, "Fault Lines," 65f.

3. See her description of the linkages between smuggled drugs, pharmaceuticals, and profiteering and the application of substandard drugs in South Asian markets in Nordstrom, "Fault Lines," 71f.

4. Stanley Cohen, *States of Denial: Knowing about Atrocities and Suffering* (Cambridge, UK: Polity, 2001); cited in Nordstrom, "Fault Lines," 80.

5. Nordstrom, "Fault Lines," 81–82.

6. Srikant Sarangi's leadership at Cardiff has generated the Centre's journal *Communication & Medicine* and an annual interdisciplinary Communication, Medicine, and Ethics conference. Ulla Connor's direction at IUPUI is a promising initiative that explores intercultural communication, an area crucially relevant in healthcare.

7. Wen-Shing Tseng and Jon Streltzer, *Cultural Competence in Health Care: A Guide for Professionals* (New York: Springer, 2008), 12.

8. Emmanuel Levinas, *Humanism of the Other*, trans. Nidra Poller (Urbana: University of Illinois Press, 2006), 18.

9. This appears distinct from Cassirer's insistence that meaning lies imbedded in culture in such a way that suggests an absolute quality to culture.

10. Desiccating both culture and tradition through reification further lends itself to exploitation of our idea of culture. Ohnuki-Tierney gives a fascinating account of this exploitation through militarizing the Japanese cultural symbol of *sakura*, cherry blossom. See Emiko Ohnuki-Tierney, *Kamikaze, Cherry Blossoms, and Nationalism: The Militarization of Aesthetics in Japanese History* (Chicago: University of Chicago Press, 2002). See also Geertz's landmark studies on the meanings of culture in Clifford Geertz, *The Interpretation of Cultures* (New York: Basic Books, 1973) and his *Available Light: Anthropological Reflections on Philosophical Topics* (Princeton, NJ: Princeton University Press, 2000).

11. Actually, there are books out there along these lines. I remember taking the Harlem Line to Manhattan from Hartsdale, NY, sitting next to a well-dressed Japanese businessman reading this sort of book in Japanese. Upon letting me look over the book, I found all sorts of common, small talk expressions on safe subjects ranging from greetings to sports, all to break the ice.

12. During a fellowship stay in Japan to study views of heart transplants and brain death, I well remember my friend and colleague Akira Akabayashi, who directs Tokyo University's Center for Biomedical Ethics and Law, offering me sage counsel in not making direct eye contact with students, professionals, and others in my seminars, particularly females as this would be construed as a sign of disrespect and even, for some, a sexual invitation. Conditioned as I am to look squarely into the eyes of one with whom I speak, I found it challenging to make the adjustment.

13. Tseng and Streltzer, *Cultural Competence in Health Care*, 13.

14. Margaret Lock, *Twice Dead: Organ Transplants and the Reinvention of Death* (Berkeley: University of California Press, 2002).

15. H. Tristram Englehardt, Jr., ed., *Global Bioethics: The Collapse of Consensus* (Salem, MA: M & M Scrivener Press, 2006).

16. Englehardt, *Global Bioethics*, 3.

17. Zygmunt Bauman, *Culture in a Liquid Modern World* (Cambridge, UK: Polity, 2011).

18. The term "cultural humility" is used in Melanie Tervalon and Jann Murray-García, "Cultural Humility Versus Cultural Competence: A Critical Distinction in Defining Physician Training Outcomes in Multicultural Education," *Journal of Health Care for the Poor and Underserved*, 9, 2, May 1998: 117–25. Also see Sayantani DasGupta, "Narrative Humility," in *Lancet*, 371, March 22, 2008: 980–81.

19. Henk ten Have, "Principlism: A Western European Appraisal," in *A Matter of Principles? Ferment in U.S. Bioethics*, eds. E.R. Du Bose, R. Hamel, and L.J. O'Connell (Valley Forge, PA: Trinity Press International, 1994): 106.

20. Levinas, *Humanism of the Other*, 25.

21. Apologies for adding another acronym to our already endless array. Acronyms have a way of short-circuiting sufficient understanding of a complex level of association. Shortcuts are not in themselves better routes to comprehension, yet our culture thrives on shortcuts, education becoming a more glaring example of the shortcut fallacy where taking the easier route via digital technologies and the like, though more entertaining, replaces the harder task of thinking critically about complex ideas. Educators who are zealous cheerleaders of these shortcuts betray their profession.

22. A landmark study is by the Institute of Medicine of the National Academies, Brian D. Smedley, Adrienne Y. Stith, and Alan R. Nelson, eds., *Unequal Treatment: Confronting Racial and Ethnic Disparities in Health Care* (Washington, DC: The National Academies Press, 2002).

23. Antonella Surbone, "Cultural Aspects of Communication in Cancer Care," *Recent Results in Cancer Research*, 168:91–104; also cited in Tseng and Streltzer, *Cultural Competence in Health Care*, 16.

24. I describe this link between cultural competency and organizational ethics in more detail in Michael C. Brannigan, "Connecting the Dots in Cultural Competency: Institutional Strategies and Conceptual Caveats," *Cambridge Quarterly of Healthcare Ethics*, 17, 2008: 173–84.

25. See M. Leininger and M.R. MacFarland, eds., *Transcultural Nursing: Concepts, Theories, Research and Practice*, 3rd ed. (New York: McGraw-Hill, 2002); J. Cioffi, "Nurses Experiences of Caring for Culturally Diverse Patients in an Acute Care Setting," *Contemporary Nurse*, 20, 2005:78–86; Nancy Crigger, Michael Brannigan, and Martha Baird, "Compassionate Nursing Professionals as Good Citizens of the World," *Advances in Nursing Science*, 29, 1, January 2006: 15–26; Nancy Crigger and Lygia Holcomb, "Practical Strategies for Providing Culturally Sensitive, Ethical Care in Developing Nations," *Journal of Transcultural Nursing*, 18, 1, January 2007: 70–76.

26. D. Ekintumas, "Nursing in Thailand: Western Concepts vs. Thai Tradition," *International Nursing Review*, 46, 1999: 55–57; cited in Tseng and Streltzer, *Cultural Competence in Health Care*, 18.

27. See Arthur Kleinman, *Patients and Healers in the Context of Culture: An Exploration of the Borderland between Anthropology, Medicine, and Psychiatry* (Berkeley: University of California Press, 1980), and his *The Illness Narratives: Suffering, Healing, and the Human Condition* (New York: Basic Books, 1988).

28. This goes hand in hand with the more traditional aspects of Islamic medicine and its four humor theory of the etiology of illness, that imbalance among the four humors—black bile, blood, phlegm, and yellow bile (associated respectively with dryness, heat, cold, and moisture)—generates illness so that restoration of balance restores health as well as enables performance of one's religious duties as prescribed in the Five Pillars. See Anahid Dervartanian Kulwicki, "People of Arab Heritage," in *Transcultural Health Care: A Culturally Competent Approach*, 2nd ed., ed. Larry D. Purnell and Betty J. Paulanka (Philadelphia: F.A. Davis Company, 2003): 90–105.

29. Though I addressed this question 15 years ago in Michael Brannigan, "Designing Ethicists," *Health Care Analysis*, 4 (1996): 206–18, to my knowledge it has evoked little response among the burgeoning congress of official "ethicists."

30. Along these lines, my colleague Wayne Shelton at the Alden March Bioethics Institute, Albany Medical College, is one scholar who is seriously examining background and core competency requirements for hospital ethics consultants. With the growing crop of ethics consultants, there is a genuine need for more studies like this.

31. While there is surely value in PowerPoint classes, these ought to supplement, not replace, in-class, interpersonal, sustained and critical discussion and dialogue, with in-depth exposure to moral reasoning and moral theory. When the supplement replaces critical analysis and face-to-face discourse, understanding can be superficial at best.

32. Renée C. Fox and Judith P. Swazey, *Observing Bioethics* (Oxford: Oxford University Press, 2008). Fox and Swazey offer an insightful narrative of the rise of bioethics within its broader sociocultural context, a must-read especially for all engaged in healthcare ethics and bioethics.

33. Paul Farmer, "Blog from the Mountains of Northern Rwanda," Team Heart Text, at http://teamhearttext.blogspot.com/, accessed 22 Feb. 2011.

34. Lock, *Twice Dead*, 11.

35. This helps explain the increasing interest in phenomenologists such as Maurice Merleau-Ponty throughout my meetings with health scholars and philosophers in Morioka, Japan.

36. Lock elaborates on the power of these "styles of reasoning" in relation to the fact/value distinction in Lock, *Twice Dead*, 32ff.

Chapter Three

Cultural Discourse and Its Hurdles

The young newlywed Kasingas left their native home in Togo, Africa, to settle in Seattle, Washington. A year later, Fauziy Kasinga gave birth to a healthy baby girl, Azinza. Just before Azinza reached her first birthday, her parents requested that she undergo a cliterodectomy, or female circumcision, at the local hospital. The hospital staff and officials adamantly opposed the request. The Kasingas then threatened to have Azinza circumcised outside of the hospital. Hospital staff and officials suspected that this would probably be under conditions that would not be sterile, and would most likely harm their baby daughter and cause serious health problems. What should the hospital authorities do?

* * *

The Japanese government does not officially recognize brain-death as the legal criterion for death. Forty-seven-year-old Akio recently moved with his family to Pittsburgh, Pennsylvania. Involved in a fatal car accident, he was pronounced brain-dead at a nearby hospital. Akio was maintained on ventilator support until his family arrived at the hospital, whereupon the neurologist indicated to them that he was clinically brain-dead. Due to their own cultural beliefs, they refused to accept the diagnosis and insisted that he be "kept alive." Out of respect for his family's wishes, and hoping that they would soon accept his death, the medical staff maintained Akio on ventilator support. As weeks went by, his family insisted that he be kept "alive." At the same time, it was evident that the ventilator could be used for other patients. His case was then presented for review by the hospital ethics committee. How should the committee go about resolving the issue?

* * *

A facility for cultural discourse in terms of basic conversation is a necessary though not sufficient ground for cultural competence. Though not equivalent to dialogue, discourse remains its precondition. Dialogue leads to mutual growth through interaction, which in its most genuine form is through face-to-face, interpersonal engagement, whereas discourse is a starting point, a conversation that requires a shared disposition, openness, language, and exchange of ideas, feelings, and perspectives. Discourse guarantees neither dialogue nor cultural competency. Nonetheless, reasoned discourse in ongoing, dynamic ways remains a necessary, vital component in cultural competency. At the same time, such discourse faces conceptual and practical barriers that need to be overcome, hurdles that are neither isolated nor compartmentalized from each other, but interpenetrate in vibrant, far-reaching, and negative fashion. Unless we properly address and work to overcome these hurdles, individual, collective, and institutional efforts to cultivate cultural competence will fall radically short of their goal.

HURDLES

Self-Referentialism

We quite naturally construct viewpoints through our own subjective lens. When we presume our viewpoints as intrinsically valid and thereby the *only* compelling point of reference, we commit the error of self-referentialism. The notion of autonomy in terms of private, individualized self-determination seems fitting within our own U.S. cultural contours. When cultural perspectives appear to clash with this understanding, we may presume our sense of autonomy to be the proper one and justify strategies to somehow encourage and convince the Other to adopt our viewpoint. In this conversion strategy, we may misguidedly consider that the Other simply lacks a sense of autonomy and moral rights. In this rather solipsistic worldview as Western biomedical missionaries, while we assign an objectivity to autonomy, by way of self-referentialism we confine ourselves within our own subjectivism. More to the point, while autonomy literally refers to "self-rule," varying views of "self," ranging from strictly individualized and private to thoroughly relational, clearly underscore divergent ways "self-rule" may be understood and applied.

Insights from Emmanuel Levinas are especially instructive. In revisiting Jean-Paul Sartre's question regarding how the self as *pour-soi*, projecting meaning, can communicate with any degree of authenticity with others, those outside the self, he reminds us of the connection between ontology and ethics. Is the self ultimately condemned to its solitude? Or is there possibility of genuine rapport in the encounter with the Other?[1] How can we avoid solipsism if each person essentially construes his or her own meaning?

In building a cultural knowledge base, we learn that due to extraordinarily far-reaching Confucian influence quite a few Asian cultures think of "self" within the relational web of family, workplace, and other significant collective matrices. I was born in Japan, and our family eventually moved to the U.S. If we had stayed in Japan, forms of address among my siblings would take into account birth order, so that I would address my younger sister as *imōto*, younger brother as *otōto*, and respectfully address my mother as *okā-san* and my father as *otō-san*, respectively meaning "younger sister," "younger brother," "honorable mother," and "honorable father." I would address them in view of their relation and roles to me. As to my relatives outside of the immediate family, it is not unusual to situate the relative within a specific locale instead of using personal names. I would allude to my Uncle Fujiya who lives in Fukuoka as *Fukuoka no oji* ("uncle in Fukuoka"). Here, language thereby depicts persons not as private entities but as immersed in a relationality that is both temporal (as in ranking siblings) and spatial (as in localizing relatives). Indeed, the most significant philosophical problem in Japanese society today has to do with this natural link between ontology and ethics and reconciling adaptations and versions of a Western emphasis upon the individual as a unique entity with the longstanding Japanese view of the individual within a web of relationality. By contrast, for us Americans who are becoming increasingly isolated as private individuals, comprehending this relational perspective becomes all the more challenging. Regardless, we stand in urgent need to seriously consider the moral merits of a relational perspective. All is not lost here, as there are prominent contemporary intellectual voices from Alisdair MacIntyre to Charles Taylor and Amitai Etzioni that underscore this relationality in various ways.[2]

Regarding what's at stake in cultural competency, one way to at least minimize self-referentialism is to consider cultural competency as an exercise in *intercultural* rather than *cross-cultural* awareness and reflection. This is not merely a matter of semantics. The danger in contemplating cultural competency as a cross-cultural exercise is that "cross-cultural" implies some secure point of reference from which we can look "across" at other cultures to assess their validity on the grounds of our own unexamined premises and, in the process, evaluate and judge another worldview strictly through the lens of our own. "Intercultural" (whether or not it succeeds the jury is still out) at least tries to break out of this referential pull, conceiving the exercise more on the basis of *parity with*, not an *overseeing of*, the Other.

In all this, culture offers an ontological and epistemological tool as a path to the Essential within that culture. For this reason, U.S. bioethics' revered tabernacle of the four principles of Autonomy, Beneficence, Nonmaleficence, and Justice, while posed as a useful set of axioms to help guide moral decision making, are also used by many in ways that transpose, or worse impose, their validity upon a culture's particularity. As Fox and Swazey point out, bioethics as it has developed has unfortunately and pretentiously assumed normative validity to universalism in the belief that some over-arching universal moral principles permeate cultures, whether or not cultures acknowledge the same. These principles as "norms that all morally serious persons share as the common morality" thus lay claim to an unspecific Ur-morality as the ground for further systematic moral construction. [3]

Yet these principles are themselves expressions of their specific culture. Through the veneer of transcending concreteness, they nonetheless presume to occupy a privileged point of reference, the assumption behind which re-grettably accompanies a "cross-cultural" framework of understanding, as a "crossing over" from one culture to another and thus from the former's vantage point. Instead, "intercultural" more naturally conveys our imbedded-ness without assigning any moral high ground to the imbedded. Once a privileged reference point assumes dominance, it becomes imperialist, cultu-rally and morally. This is not to deny clear practical benefits to the four principle approach. It offers a coherent, cohesive typology and template, a lucid menu with spelled out conceptual and theoretical items with which to apply to extremely complex and untidy situations. It is a case's untidiness that unsettles us. Yet, the formulae can too neatly simplify. Indeed, both Thomas Beauchamp and James Childress, who author the classic text *Princi-ples of Biomedical Ethics*, warn us of the dangers in such reductionist appli-cation. [4] The authority of principles belies a triumph in reductionism and, moreover, satisfies presuppositions regarding some transcendent, universal moral order that surpasses particularity.

Homogenization

As a first commandment in intercultural studies, *Thou shalt not cast mono-lithic nets over cultures*. Net-casting ignores both meaningful internal varia-tions and external correspondence with other cultures. [5] For example, first-generation Mexican immigrants in California may rightfully assert their dif-ferences from second, third, and so on generations. Indeed, there may be more intra-cultural distinctions than inter-cultural. As in Japanese *Nihonjin-ron*, classifying a culture as homogenous and exceptional is not only mistak-en but leads to pernicious patterns of simplification and skewed cultural discourse. Although most Chinese are Han, the rest comprise numerous na-tionalities and ethnic groupings. The Chinese culture remains intensely com-plex and not prone to easy generalizations. [6] Furthermore, although Mandarin is the official language, it has ten different dialects, and Chinese themselves have difficulty understanding the different dialects.

Asian patients can come from a variety of Asian backgrounds, each with their specific and unique cultures (China, Japan, Korea, Southeast Asia, and so on). Here, homogenization is particularly pernicious when reasonable generalization gives way to stereotyping that polarizes groups, bifurcating a complex culture and bundle of sub-cultures like stereotyping Asians as collective-oriented and interdependent *in contrast* to Westerners. Nonetheless, here we need to seek a necessary balance between acknowledging certain general tendencies (Asians tend to be interdependent rather than private and independent) and recognizing distinctions (more Asians are exerting self-expression and individuality on various levels).[7] Homogenization is an all-too-common fallacy in cultural discourse that spawns a hazardous reductionism. Confucian thought does not refute the existence of individual, unique persons and individuality. Nor does Confucianism principally view the individual being *per se* as an independent entity of the type emphasized throughout a good portion of Western intellectual thought. Cultural competency studies that offer a bullet-point shopping list of cultural features risk these sorts of misleading inaccuracies.

Bear in mind that generalizations remain distinct from homogenization as the latter molds generalizations into an inflexible catalog of traits and one-dimensional packaging of a complex culture. We generalize when we understand that African Americans undeniably suffer particularly from hypertension disorders, much of which stems from factors including high sodium intake, high blood pressure, weight issues combined with a sedentary lifestyle, and stress. As a group, they tend to be genetically prone to sickle-cell anemia and high glucose, and they have the highest incidence among ethnic groups of HIV/AIDS.[8] Our generalizing signals a natural need to understand a group as a group, to somehow grasp a group's identity through detecting specific patterns prevalent within that group. Yet homogenizing African-Americans wraps them all under a blanket of sameness. While a quick snapshot of Hindus, Muslims, and Jews regarding dietary strictures has its practical benefits, according to one study in cultural competency, Buddhists are vegetarians who "consider all living beings that can move around as *having a soul*, and the killing of them is forbidden" (author italics).[9] Granted, many if not most Buddhists (at least the many I know) do not eat meat. Yet a fundamental tenet in Buddhist teachings is that of *anatta* ("no self" or "no soul"). Orthodox Buddhist teachings refute the idea that we are independent selves or souls (the Hindu *atman*) separate from all others. *Anatta* (Sanskrit, *anatman*) is for Buddhists one of the three signs of existence, the other two being *dukkha* (suffering) and *anicca* (impermanence). Readers of the above misconstrual can easily fail to see Buddhism's unique distinction from Hindu and other faith traditions regarding individual identity, self, and soul.

Reification

Reification is the use of certain terms and ideas that are by their nature dynamic in an objectified fashion so that the referent of such terms and phrases is considered thing-like. In casting this fixed, thing-like quality to the referent, defined within tight and rigid boundaries, we stultify an idea or term that is vital and alive. This type of plundering is prevalent, often undetected, and without accountability. Reifying is the perfect epistemological crime that negates the dynamic quality of the referent.

When it comes to cultural comparison, we often reify the notion of "culture" by all too easily succumbing to cultural tags. These may offer easy explanations, but are generally misleading. "Culture" is often a seductive panacea that hides an enormously complex bundle of factors among which socio-cultural considerations are simply one feature among many. Uncritically resorting to "culture" is especially misleading when we associate "culture" strictly with "tradition," the latter often considered to contrast what is "modern" and "secular" and thus viewed on that account as antiquated, even archaic. Consider the use of historical descriptors like "traditional" in opposition to "modern." Our conceptions of particular cultures are generally historically glued, so that unless we have a specific historical period in mind, these terms are vague at best. Notions of "traditional" cultures may thereby evoke varying images of an obscure past connoting, for example, some nostalgic golden age versus a corrupt "modern" era. Furthermore, by reifying "culture" and "tradition," either term becomes prey to political exploitation as in misconceptions surrounding Islamic culture or Muslim tradition. Here, both "culture" and "tradition" can be used as rhetorical tools. To illustrate, Japanese opposition to brain death, though often reduced to culture, encompasses other factors including a steadily increasing climate of public distrust in the medical profession, such distrust resulting from a series of notorious scandals like the Juro Wada affair in 1968 following Japan's first heart transplant in which a heart was extracted under highly suspicious circumstances. For nearly 30 years after this scandal, the Japanese officially prohibited heart transplants.[10] Reifying "culture" abstracts from a dynamic, real lived experience and totalizes it without recognizing subtle though powerful forces. No doubt, distrust in physicians stands out given a long-standing cultural tradition of deference and respect for professional authority. Rather than static, the notion of culture is fluid with changing, shifting undercurrents.

There are palpable errors in reifying, for example, "African culture" or "African tradition" particularly since exaggerating the role of "culture" when attempting to fathom the perspective of the Other sanctions us to be less prone to critically examine our own perspectives. Many Muslim patients and their families tend to resist end-of-life advance planning and decision-making for various reasons, including ultimate trust and faith in the will of Allah, and traditional deference to the authority of the physician. To naively bundle their objection to this type of discussion as simply "cultural" short-circuits us from reexamining our own presuppositions regarding end of life deliberations.

In similar measure, we often reify our sense of "rights" and view them as representing some given entity that we claim as our own. More precisely, what does it mean when we claim to have a "right" to x? What lies beneath the surface of the claim? Reifying settles for the surface rather than digging deeper to uncover distinctions along the way involving a variety of contexts—human, animal, moral, legal, constitutional, civic, individual, collective, cultural, and so on. Enwrapped in the glamour of non-distinction, we've lost interest in distinctions.[11] When we more closely examine the nature of, for example, moral rights as distinct from legal, further archeology unearths conceptual and practical distinctions in view of moral rights' relation to duties, entitlements, positive and negative moral rights, and the all-unsettling question regarding universality and relativism, in the process discovering how our own cultural gestalt constructs our constructing. For instance, prior to the Meiji Restoration, no Japanese term came close to what we refer to as a "right," whether moral or legal. In 1868, to accommodate Western pressure, the newly formulated term *kenri*, combining *ken* ("power") and *ri* ("principle" and "interest") and meaning the "principle or interest of power" associated with persons, though aiming to be equivalent to our Western term, still falls short of our understanding of "right."

In cultural competency work, the acquisition of a knowledge base of specific cultures risks weak comparisons when drawing inferences on the grounds of either presence or absence of certain terms. The absence of a proper or sufficient enough term for "right" in the Japanese language does not necessarily infer an absence of "right" as we conceive of it. Terms need to be understood within their specific cultural and historical contexts so that in matters of linguistic assistance in an institution's cultural competency strategy, fluency requires more than transliteral knowledge of another language. Absent contextual understanding of how terms and ideas elicit their essential dynamic quality, we fall prey to reification.

Measurability Bias

A major hurdle lies in Western biomedicine's bias towards measurability and quantifiability as *the* unquestioned standard for what is real. We increasingly identify "value" in terms of measurability and "medical" with measurable. Enamored by new and sophisticated medical technologies, we place more confidence in the device itself which assumes its own hegemony by virtue of its "objectifiability," a dominion of technical intervention that subordinates human interaction and interpretation. In the U.S. especially, the deeper issue here lies in how we humans relate to our tools. Reliance on our devices can lead to our devices using us, and in turn we ourselves becoming devices of our tools. As we've suggested, for all its life-saving wonders, assumptions underlying organ transplantation may dissociate "person" from body, reflecting an increasing depersonalization of the human as merely a body and its attendant parts so that vital organs become mere commodities.[12] Margaret Lock reminds us of Marx's critique of capitalism's inevitably churning out a "fetishism of commodities," bestowing intrinsic value to the commodity itself as object *sans* context. Indeed for consumers, that all-important relational, social, economic, historical, and political context *behind* the commodity, the process which leads to the final glimmering product, is disregarded, abandoned, ignored. Walk through any mall, and we witness decontextualized final products, end results, without their history. Applying Stanley Cohen's knowledge/acknowledge distinction, we know the product yet disacknowledge its temporal and historic lineage.

In effect, measurability represents our singular contemporary ailment, "sin," our socio-cultural "evil" if we defer to Paul Ricouer's sense of evil as "missing the mark"—our prevailing acontextualization, the recognition of which is all too demanding, requiring perspective, historical understanding, and situational comprehension. Abandoning context naturally commodifies, commodification denoting reification's sibling. Viewing the patient as a mere occupant of a bed warranting specific here-and-now treatment modalities until discharge according to a payment per diem schedule transforms the patient as person into patient as commodity. In the process, just as we disregard what is behind each commodity, we overlook the profound question— What is behind the patient? To which the answer is: a complex narrative that we *must* somehow tap into while also admitting our fallibility in truly knowing the patient, the stranger, in his or her entirety. More phenomenologically, as with any object of our perception the patient remains *en soi pour moi*, "in itself for me." As *en soi*, in himself and herself, the patient transcends us in that he or she goes well beyond my limited understanding. The patient is forever a mystery as distinct from a "problem," problem denoting some puzzle that has a solution and a mystery as impenetrable, unknowable. As *pour moi*, the patient reveals him- or herself to me for me to address. The patient's presence solicits my presence.

Normalizing Discourse

There is a normalizing quality to cultural discourse that can lead to imprudent reflection and thinking. "Language is a loaded gun," says Dwight Bollinger. Careless thinking in particular comes about under the canon of the "what if" scenario, one that evokes a prevailing mind set which is less critical and more bifurcated. Philosophical thought experiments, all too common and often useful, inspire deliberation in order to test the limits of moral theory in general, such as utilitarianism, and specific rules and application in particular. Yet a thought experiment ought to be on a par with what is realistically plausible, not constructed purely out of fantasy. Reality, not fantasy, should test limits of moral theory, the realm of oughtness. Reality, not fantasy, is the ground for the normative. How we ought to act can only be properly situated in what is practically (less than conceptually) possible. What we *ought* to do can only be grounded in what we *can* do.

To illustrate, consider the perplexing questions surrounding the morality of torture in the "ticking bomb" scenario, typically described as follows.[13] The FBI has seized a suspect who is believed to know the whereabouts of a ticking bomb about to explode in a public area within an hour or two. As interrogation goes nowhere, interrogators, now growing desperate for information, propose torture, ranging from mild to severe, as an option, torture conventionally defined as:

> any act by which severe pain or suffering, whether physical or mental, is intentionally inflicted on a person for such purposes as obtaining from that person or a third person information or confession, punishing that person for an act committed or suspected to have been committed, or intimidating or dehumanizing that person or other persons.[14]

This scenario is usually framed in the form of an either/or proposition: either torture in this case is justified or it is not. Arguments are then raised routinely in the form of conflicting moral theories. Opponents, groups like the World Medical Association, the Tokyo Declaration, Amnesty International, Red Cross, Human Rights Watch, and Physicians for Human Rights, often apply deontological grounds for their prohibition. Defenders of torture in this situation, on the other hand, such as the Landau Commission in its defense of "moderate physical pressure," the U.S. in its notion of "exceptional interrogational techniques," and Alan Dershowitz with his "necessity defense" often resort to utilitarian theory. Posing the scenario in this fashion may nicely analyze and deconstruct moral theories. However, framing the problem in this way is itself simplistic and dangerously naïve. Digging further into the situation, questions of intent, means, effectiveness, and time necessarily enter in. For instance, as to the interrogated, what does he know? How will he be interrogated? And what about the plaguing issue of agency? Who interrogates? And to turn utilitarianism on its head, what about long-term consequences for the state, society, and meanings bestowed to human dignity?

In similar fashion, we often encounter an uncritical use of what we label as a "moral (or ethical) dilemma," an all too familiar mantra in hospital ethics committee discourse, healthcare conferences, symposia, courses, literature, cases, all pointing to some moral catch-22 in which we are forced to choose between the lesser of two evils. The "necessary evil" syndrome. Yet, in any given scenario, the "ought" can only be grounded in the plausible and practically possible. Therefore, this gives pause to reconsider whether what is framed as a moral dilemma is indeed a genuine moral dilemma. Or is it rather a dilemma that is logistic and practical, like rescuing two persons from a burning building, each person at far ends of the conflagration, and it is impossible to rescue both. In which case this constitutes a practical dilemma rather than a moral one.

At least in theory, a moral dilemma occurs in a situation which calls for a set of moral duties that are incompatible with each other since they cannot be performed at the same time. I may have a moral duty to do x and y. However, I cannot do both. Doing x precludes me from performing y. Immanuel Kant's classic formula is apropos:

> A *conflict of duties* (*collision officiorum s. obligationum*) would be a relation of duties in which one of them would annul the other (wholly or in part). But a *conflict of duties* and obligations is inconceivable (*obligations non colliduntur*). For the concepts of duty and obligation as such express the objective practical *necessity* of certain actions, and two conflicting rules cannot both be necessary at the same time. [15]

Moral dilemmas are themselves irresolvable, whereas it is entirely possible to resolve a moral conflict, tension, or problem. In a moral conflict, it is not a matter of being morally obliged to do *both* x and y, but one *or* the other. My moral duty to be honest with my patient and to disclose his prognosis may conflict with my moral duty to respect his prior request to not be so informed, in which case I need to determine which duty trumps the other, and I feel morally justified in honoring his prior request. Not all philosophers agree with this assessment of moral dilemmas. Ruth Barcan Marcus offers persuasive arguments for the existence of moral dilemmas. [16] In her analysis, moral dilemmas are indeed real and she poses the example of having to save one identical twin when both lives are in danger and circumstances preclude saving both. For Marcus, though a Kantian "ought" rests upon a "can," one cannot presume universally embraced interpretations of both "ought" and "can."

Arguments like this continue to debate the possibility or impossibility of a genuine moral dilemma. The point here is that the issue remains controversial, while bioethics discourse avoids any hint of debate, and in uncritically presuming the *de facto* existence of moral dilemmas does little to distinguish between moral dilemma and moral conflict. The unexamined rubric in bioethics conveys the idea that moral dilemmas are undeniably rampant.

ON COLLABORATION AND AGREEMENT

So how can we sufficiently address the reality of diverse and colliding world-views? Here, the noteworthy insights of Tristram Englehardt deserve further commentary. He goes so far as to claim that moral pluralism represents a system of underlying metaphysical, epistemological, and socio-cultural rifts, or, as I put it, deep-rooted fault lines, that essentially minimizes if not prohibits altogether any possibility of resolution. All truths become context-derivative, not reflecting some objective, transcendent reality. For Englehardt, we are trapped within our own subjectivities, "at best within intersubjectivity" so that truth is "multiple." [17]

The result is that there is no longer truth in the sense of an independent reality to be known, or at least an independent moral reality, but instead all truths become interpretations within the hermeneutic of a particular moral narrative. [18]

Since Englehardt finds no rationally persuasive grounds upon which to assert some universal moral bioethics, he argues that the best we can hope for is collaborative negotiation and agreement:

> [T]here is no universal, rationally justifiable, moral perspective, or even common notion of the reasonable that could provide the basis for deliberative democratic polities or their governance. Instead, there are at best procedural modes of collaboration that allow negotiation and limited agreement, as in the markets. [19]

This presses upon us our first prerogative—not imposing *our* truth, but directing our critical gaze more upon *how* we deliberate with each other within the context of moral diversity. For Englehardt, this requires that we:

> recognize procedural means for working together in the face of moral and metaphysical disagreement. This strategy binds those separated by different moral and metaphysical visions, who draw their authority from neither God nor Reason, but from common agreement. This immanent approach affirms as the heuristic and exemplar model for moral investigation and collaboration, the image of the market, a moral space where free and responsible individuals can through agreement venture together in limited enterprises. [20]

In which case, the "market," in terms of free exchange of ideas, becomes for Englehardt a "heuristic" model of peaceful collaboration and agreement.

To all this I offer a two-layered response. First, Englehardt's choice above of the term "intersubjectivity" is puzzling. True, we act as individual, separate "subjects," approximating a Leibnizian sense of self as separate monads. I would argue that this is especially the case today despite our claims to enhanced connectivity. For *connectivity*—the increasing fact of our networked lives—does not capture the essence of *connectedness*, that is, genuine interrelation, engagement, the heart of which lies in what I describe in the next chapter as "presence." "Intersubjectivity," however, following Englehardt's logic, is not the best term. The prefix, *inter*, gives it away for the same reason I favor "intercultural" over "cross-cultural." While the latter suggests some privileged point of reference from which we "cross over" to examine, inspect, converse with, and possibly impose our perspective, *inter* entails the more hopeful, perhaps idealistic, possibility of putting aside (as in a phenomenological *epoché* or bracketing) our natural bias (particularly metaphysical and epistemological) in order to collaborate with some measure of open-minded sensitivity and reasonableness. Therefore intersubjectivity is more demanding than Englehardt allows. Intersubjectivity (as in the spirit of Gabriel Marcel and Martin Buber) requires that we transcend our isolated, monadic subjectivity, or "I," *in order to* engage more authentically with *other subjects*, other "I"s, not as objects for scrutiny, manipulation, or exploitation, but as subjects, as "Thou"s in the case of Buber, with their own distinct visions and worldviews. It is precisely this intersubjectivity that undergirds inter-presence, a being to, for, and with others. As I later argue, embodied presence and inter-presence, denoting connectedness, is its own truth.

My second layer of concern lies in Englehardt's use of "market" as a heuristic model for peaceable collaboration. While on its most basic level, market refers to a free exchange of ideas, a marketplace of discourse, it too stands in danger of becoming another privileged reference point once we extract "free" from market. Realistically, not all have access to the market. Not all have the power and the means to provide services for exchange in the market. So also, not all can participate in the free exchange of discourse. Nonetheless, through Englehardt's description of this market as a "moral space where free and responsible individuals can through agreement venture together in limited enterprises," Englehardt regards "peaceable collaboration" as a default position in view of fundamental moral differences, and he further asserts that this "peaceable collaboration is understood as to involve the eschewal of coercion against the unconsenting innocent. The notion of peaceable interaction does not preclude employing justified punitive or defensive force."[21]

His analysis occurs within the context of his view of the fundamental exclusivity of two conflicting moral visions. The first is that of a universal moral perspective rationally constructed through universal notions of freedom and justice. Here, theories of justice comprise a menu from which we can select a Rawlsian "original position," a Kantian principle of universalizability, or a Millian principle of utility and the greater good, all theories that assume a right action grounded upon some universal moral standards. In this first vision, a "universal social democratic framework" works to accommodate moral pluralism so that it fits into its universalist scheme. On the other hand, Englehardt's "libertarian framework" underscores a moral pluralism whose participants share common ground through peaceable collaboration in the market of ideas, and protected from state coercion. This position is enriched through the metaphor of market, absent some universal moral standard, as a "moral trading floor, a space within which peaceable, consenting moral agents can frame joint projects with willing others."[22]

Again, is this market model an appropriate enough metaphor if analogous to the Western trading market where trading power remains a decisive factor in trade eligibility? Amidst the ruckus of bartering among digital power-holders like Verizon, AT&T, Time-Warner, and so on in the marketing of our 'vital organs' of connectivity—mobile phones, laptops, iPhones, and more, where are those voices representing poor and destitute Americans in rural areas as well as inner cities who, because they cannot afford such devices, are at an unfair disadvantage without access to online services, such access held as the social norm? Digging deeper, where are those voices representing the young children in the Democratic Republic of Congo who mine coltan, that vital mineral without which we wouldn't have our "necessities"? Those on the trading floor may be "peaceable and consenting moral agents," but other voices are left out, excluded, and remain invisible. We traders on the floor are not present to those absent. As Zygmunt Bauman puts it, as market forces are subjected to and sustained through power plays and consequential disparities and inequities, we remain "indifferent to difference." In fact, Bauman deftly describes how the infectious sway of globalization and its various market strategies feed a thriving ethos of consumerism, sustained by power imbalances that persist not only despite but *on account of saccharin calls for respecting cultural diversity under the rubric of "multiculturalism."* He notes the duplicity that breeds our "indifference to difference," that is, real difference in terms of glaring material poverty:

> The new indifference to difference presents itself in theory as an approval of 'cultural pluralism': the political practice formed and supported by this theory is defined by the term 'multiculturalism.' It is apparently inspired by the postulate of liberal tolerance and of support for communities' rights to independence and to public acceptance of their chosen (or inherited) identities. In reality, however, it acts as a socially conservative force. Its achievement is the transformation of social inequality, a phenomenon highly unlikely to win general approval, into the guise of 'cultural diversity.' . . . Through this linguistic measure, the moral ugliness of poverty magically turns, as if by the touch of a fairy's wand, into the aesthetic appeal of cultural diversity . . . calls for the respect of cultural differences bring little comfort to the many communities that are *deprived of the power of independence by virtue of their handicap, and doomed to have their 'own' choices made by other, more substantial powers.*"[23] (author italics)

Appealing to a market image thus belies a particularist vision that assumes a "market" model as universal. In a sense, Englehardt hints at this when he points out that peaceable collaboration requires our capacity to coexist and collaborate without coercion. Nonetheless, his market model discounts the ineluctable force of power structures that are institutional and systemic, a regrettable feature of our collective human condition yet inevitable without principles and rules to encourage equity. If we rely merely on a peaceable collaboration as our default posture in the face of moral disagreement, we passively acquiesce to moral incongruities that, in my view, reinforce and sustain unnecessary suffering of other living beings. In this regard, the Buddhist call to relieve suffering remains a universal moral imperative. It could be argued, for instance, that regardless of how we rank what Englehardt offers as the four overriding concerns—liberty, equality, prosperity, and security[24]—they share common ground of the over-arching value and concern in the Buddhist sense of working to relieve suffering, as well as contributing to the Aristotelian notion of *eudaimonia*, or human flourishing. Surely, rankings are context-dependent, yet contextuality does not in itself annul possible shared moral visions.

Here is where Englehardt's notion of "permission" is particularly relevant. He advocates a "secular morality as a procedural framework" to enable peaceable collaboration grounded on "permission of those who choose peaceably to collaborate in acting morally."[25] As described, this idea of "permission" raises questions. As to those who "choose peaceably to collaborate," who are these who choose? Again, not all are free to choose. More vulnerable and marginalized peoples have little or no access to the privilege of choice. Along the lines of Englehardt's insightful critique of UNESCO's 2005 Declaration (mentioned in the previous chapter), are indigenous voices represented? Critics of the Human Genome Project, the international effort to map our entire human genetic makeup (initiated in 1990 in the U.S. with, by the way, only 5% of public funding allocated to examine ethical, legal, and social implications, or ELSI) pointed out that most of the human genome research was conducted on people of European descent (constituting 15% of the world population), overlooking the rest of the world. For this reason, The Human Genome Diversity Project (HGDP) was established in order to collect and examine blood samples from various indigenous groups and to thus broaden the scope of genome research. Yet even this effort generated strident criticism that the HGDP, or "vampire project," was in effect a marketing ploy to exploit select indigenous groups for biotech companies' profit. Sustained denunciation of the HGDP led to the 1993 Mataatua Declaration on Cultural and Intellectual Property Rights of Indigenous Peoples, put together by representatives from indigenous groups in Australia, New Zealand, Cook

Islands, Japan, Fiji, India, Peru, Panama, Philippines, Suriname, and the U.S., an impressive organized effort to stem the tide of corporate exploitation of indigenous peoples and their bodies as commodities. [26]

Because he discounts rational grounds for moral consensus, Englehardt's reasoning falls back on itself so that his "permission" encounters the moral pluralism and absence of universal consensus it seeks to address as a default posture. In essence, what is at issue in all this? Is there genuine incompatible moral pluralism? It is not clear why moral pluralism as a fact indicates necessary incompatibility. More basically, what is moral pluralism? If we admit that moral pluralism gives rise to moral incompatibility and thus in-commensurable positions and thereby an absence of resolution, Englehardt's default "permission" fails to escape the same pluralism and incompatibility. In which case, this, the intercultural possibility of safely crossing cultural fault lines, requires all the more an understanding of toleration, its varying degrees, and its limits.

ON TOLERANCE

Cultural competency work inevitably encounters the challenging problematic of accommodation and its limits, or what we ordinarily think of as tolerance. Awareness of and sensitivity to a multitude of culturally grounded narratives, without some conceptual orienting sense, can lead to the perplexing assump-tion that all narratives occupy the same normative level and that all are morally acceptable in various degrees. When this Sameness triumphs over Otherness questions regarding tolerance and its limits are especially acute. Problems erupt when we raise tolerance *per se* to high moral ground, virtue-like, and nearly absolute. Tolerance has its limits. [27] How far do we accom-modate the beliefs and values of Others, particularly if doing so conflicts with a health institution's mission statement? How far should Catholic hospi-tals go in informing a rape victim of options to terminate pregnancy that results from the rape? The question of tolerance is perhaps the most volatile consequence in cultural competency work. To my knowledge, this has not been sufficiently explored in the context of cultural competency. For this reason, the following brief excursus can hopefully illuminate the problematic concerning tolerance.

Surely it seems reasonable to uphold, as does Ruth Macklin, the existence of universal principles (for instance in the arena of human rights) without insisting on moral absolutism and rigidity. [28] Sensitivity to cultural interpreta-tions and applications of universal standards is not reducible to moral relati-vism. All this segues into considerations of tolerance and its limits. What we need is a sound conceptual orientation to more properly understand the meaning of tolerance. And when we inspect the idea of tolerance, we detect its imprecise nature. In cultural competency work, tolerance in principle carries wide appeal. Nonetheless, as with the concept of cultural competency, tolerance lacks philosophical precision. Bringing some further clarity to ideas of tolerance therefore is all the more imperative given our increasing awareness of apparent moral pluralism.

Tolerance essentially involves not intervening in those things about which we disapprove. In terms of John Horton's instructive analysis, tolerance therefore involves first our *objecting* to something or someone, and then our *non-interfering* despite our criticism.[29] In its bare bones, when we tolerate something or someone, we believe one way but act in another. I morally disapprove of female genital circumcision for reasons I hold to be morally relevant. If I refrain from intervening in this action in a specific circumstance, for instance in some Egyptian village where the practice is not uncommon, I tolerate the act. I would not tolerate the act in a U.S. hospital. I morally disapprove of a husband's insistence that his wife secure his permission before she consents to her own medical treatment. Should I refrain from intervening in this particular instance if I am in the Philippines where it is more common, I demonstrate tolerance. Are these two instances of tolerance of equal moral weight? Equally justifiable? The fact of disagreement as to what beliefs and actions we should accept and what we should reject and in different contexts underscores the problematic behind the notion of tolerance.

To begin with, why would I tolerate that which I find morally objectionable? If I morally object to abortion on the grounds that I believe it is the unjustified destruction of an innocent human life, why would I refrain from negatively intervening and speaking out against abortion? For this reason, Bernard Williams asserts that tolerance, though necessary, is impossible.[30] Necessary because, as Isaiah Berlin reminds us, "conflicts of value are real and inescapable, with some of them having no satisfactory solution."[31] Furthermore, there are varying degrees of moral objection. There are those instances that I may find utterly objectionable, absolutely immoral, and therefore intolerable for all sorts of reasons. There are those other actions and beliefs to which I morally object, yet the degree of my objection ranges from mild to strong, and again for various reasons I manage to tolerate and put up with them. These reasons constitute part of the complex package of tolerance. My reasons for tolerating what I believe to be morally objectionable illustrate the complexity behind the idea of tolerance. The danger in all this, however, particularly as it relates to cultural competence, is that we can avoid having to churn through this complexity by simply sliding into the comfort zone of extreme positions—either absolute tolerance, tolerating all things we morally disapprove of, or outright intolerance, tolerating nothing we morally object to. Here, striking an Aristotelian balance to avoid excessive and/or deficient tolerance is critical. Excessive tolerance not only per-mits carte blanche cultural rationalizing for what is morally legitimate but is also harmful. As Macklin states, "Although respect for cultural diversity mandates tolerance of the beliefs and practices of others, in some situations excessive tolerance can produce harm to patients."[32] Deficient tolerance, on the other hand, continues to rear its disfigured head in contemporary modes of bigotry, cultural stereotyping, and defamation of traditions different from our own. John Locke's classic view of tolerance is in the context of an absolutist prohibition of free religious expression.

Cultural competency work is particularly relevant here since it fosters a growing recognition of moral pluralism that may not only engender a fruitful awareness of diversity but also a sense of uncritical acceptance and even leading to moral indifference. If Japanese family members in an American hospital refuse to accept the determination that their son is clinically brain dead, a determination confirmed by three neurologists, do we therefore toler-ate their belief and keep their son "alive" on a ventilator, a scarce resource that could be used by other patients, in the name of cultural sensitivity and competency? Diversity awareness is a two-edged sword. There are indeed rich benefits in growing globally aware. UNESCO's "Universal Declaration on Cultural Diversity" (2002) proposes universal principles in the context of cultural diversity, an apparent attempt to reconcile tensions between univer-salism with particularism. There are clear implications for tolerance here in both principle and practice. Diversity awareness also means that behaviors that we believe are morally unjustified may become more acceptable, spur-ring a divide between the moral attitude behind tolerance and moral judg-ment, as noted by Barbara Herman:

> The demand for context-sensitive judgment leads to an awkward impasse. In conditions of deep social pluralism, the moral attitudes liberal toleration per-mits (and part of the values it supports) are inhospitable to the conditions on judgment necessary for justifying toleration. In encouraging a partition be-tween moral attitudes and moral judgment liberal toleration can be, in a practi-cal sense, self-defeating.[33]

Put simply, espousing tolerance because noninterference reflects cultural competency and sensitivity is not enough. Since tolerance consists of both *restraint* from intervening and *objection* to an action or belief, focusing solely on the matter of restraint is merely passive tolerance. If we focus solely on not intervening purely on the grounds of cultural competence, we risk ignoring the grounds of why we object in the first place. Rather than think of tolerance in its passive sense of restraint, we need to reenergize the concept by redirecting our focus to more closely examine reasons for *both* objecting and not interfering.

In the process of examining our reasons for both disapproval and restraint, we need to be aware of the critical distinction between "dislike" and "disapprove."[34] Tolerance does entail refraining from conduct one simply dislikes, though dislike usually leads to disapproval. Of course, in view of the symbiotic relationship between feeling and thinking, clearly demarcating "dislike" and "disapprove" is tricky. Feelings do play a valuable role in moral judgments. Indeed, Leon Kass argues they play a major role, for instance, with respect to gut feelings of "repugnance" we may have towards human reproductive cloning.[35] Whether or not we ought to always listen to our "gut" is arguable. Nonetheless, tolerance in the real sense hinges on objections to actions and beliefs on the basis of moral reasoning and not purely on feelings. Otherwise, by equating tolerance simply with restraint based solely on feelings, we may consider conduct intolerable when it is not. In order to properly understand tolerance, especially in the realm of cultural competency we need to critically examine our reasons for both restraint and disapproval, so that we ask: Is my objection reasonable? If so, why is it right for me to restrain? Tolerance thus has its limits. If we reduce tolerance to uncritical acceptance of a culture's beliefs, values, and practices, we step onto the shifting soil of moral relativism.

Cultural competency work needs to avoid equating cultural understanding and sensitivity with tolerating any and all of a culture's beliefs, values, and practices. Cultural respect does not infer that we embrace practices with which we disagree. We can learn to understand *why*, for instance, Togolese parents may insist upon clitoridectomy for their infant daughter, but this is a far cry from accepting it. Of course, proper evaluation can only come about as a result of proper understanding, knowing the relevant facts in their historical, cultural context. As Macklin incisively reminds us, explaining a certain practice is not the same as morally justifying it.[36] Cultural tolerance is undeniably crucial, yet it has its boundaries. Uncritical tolerance spawns a moral relativism with which cultural competency remains irreconcilable. To be sure, as a healthcare organization carries out its cultural competency efforts, it will need to confront this ongoing challenge in resolving cross-cultural conflicts.

NOTES

1. In this regard, Sartre's "Existentialism as a Humanism" fashions hope of human solidarity.

2. This helps explain why disaster scenarios are a particular source of social angst. The prospect of triaging victims of H1N1 or in any other pandemic has induced numerous commentaries, many of which underscore the intense difficulty of both triaging and rationing in a social and cultural ethos of individual, private liberties.

3. Fox and Swazey, *Observing Bioethics*, 158; see discussion in 157ff.

4. Tom L. Beauchamp and James F. Childress, *Principles of Biomedical Ethics*, 5th ed, (New York: Oxford University Press, 2011): 11ff.

5. I address net-casting further in the context of intercultural bioethics in Michael C. Brannigan, "*Ikiru* and Net-Casting in Intercultural Bioethics," in *Bioethics at the Movies*, ed. Sandra Shapshay (Baltimore, MD: The Johns Hopkins University Press, 2009): 345–65.

6. Purnell and Paulanka, *Transcultural Health Care*, 106.

7. Labeling Asians as strictly collective and solely relational is wrongheaded. It makes better sense to consider their ontologies to be more reflective of dual-identities of both individual and relational. Watsuji Tetsuro emphasizes this when he examines the natural relationship between *ningen* ("human being") and *aidagara* ("in-betweenness"). See Watsuji Tetsuro, *Rinrigaku* (Ethics in Japan), trans. Yamamoto Seisaku (Albany: State University of New York Press, 1996; orig. in Tokyo: Iwanami Shoten, Publishers, 1937). Along similar lines, the Confucian virtue *ren*, meaning humaneness and benevolence, combines the character for individual and two.

8. Tseng and Streltzer, *Cultural Competence in Health Care*, 43.

9. Tseng and Streltzer, *Cultural Competence in Health Care*, 23.

10. My article more closely looks at these other factors in Michael C. Brannigan, "A Chronicle of Organ Transplant Progress in Japan," *Transplant International*, 5 (1992): 180–86.

11. This is increasingly evident in academia in higher education with the increasingly rampant conviction of non-distinctions among disciplines, in polar opposition to purists who focus only on the distinctions.

12. There is an irony here in views regarding enhancement technologies and their effect on the relationship between body and self. See Carl Elliott, *Better than Well: American Medicine Meets the American Dream* (New York: Norton, 2003).

13. See Bob Brecker, *Torture and the Ticking Bomb* (Malden, MA: Blackwell Publishing, 2007); here he constructively exposes the fallacy behind fantasy-based thought experiments.

14. Christopher Tindale, "The Logic of Torture," *Social Theory and Practice*, 22 (1996): 355; cited in Brecker, *Torture*, 5.

15. Immanuel Kant, "Introduction to the Metaphysic of Morals," in *The Doctrine of Virtue, Part II of the Metaphysic of Morals*, trans. Mary J. Gregory (Philadelphia: University of Pennsylvania Press, 1971); cited in *Moral Dilemmas*, ed. Christopher W. Gowans (New York: Oxford University Press, 1987), 39.

16. Ruth Barcan Marcus, "Moral Dilemmas and Consistency," in Gowans, *Moral Dilemmas*, 188–204.

17. H. Tristram Englehardt, Jr., ed., *Global Bioethics: The Collapse of Consensus* (Salem, MA: M & M Scrivener Press, 2006), 16. My thanks to a reviewer's suggestion that I more closely attend to Englehardt's views on collaboration.

18. Englehardt, *Global Bioethics*, 16.

19. Englehardt, *Global Bioethics,* 8.

20. Englehardt, *Global Bioethics*, 16.

21. Englehardt, "The Search for a Global Morality: Bioethics, the Culture Wars, and Moral Diversity," in Englehardt, *Global Bioethics*, 41, note 1.

22. Englehardt, "Search for a Global Morality," 23.

23. Zygmunt Bauman, *Culture in a Liquid Modern World* (Cambridge, UK: Polity, 2011), 46.

24. Englehardt, "Search for a Global Morality," 24.

25. Englehardt, "Search for a Global Morality," 25.

26. Michael C. Brannigan and Judith A. Boss, *Healthcare Ethics in a Diverse Society* (Mountain View, CA: Mayfield Publishing Co., 2001), 254–55; The Mataatua Declaration is included on p. 255.

27. For a rich discussion, see P. Ricoeur, ed. *Tolerance between Intolerance and the Intolerable* (Providence, RI: Berghahn Books, 1996).

28. Ruth Macklin, *Against Relativism: Cultural Diversity and the Search for Ethical Universals in Medicine* (New York: Oxford University Press, 1999).

29. John Horton, "Toleration as a Virtue," in *Toleration: An Elusive Virtue*, ed. David Heyd (Princeton, NJ: Princeton University Press, 1996): 28–43.

30. Bernard Williams, "Toleration: An Impossible Virtue?" in Heyd, *Toleration*, 18–27.

31. Cited in Fox and Swazey, *Observing Bioethics*, 167.

32. Ruth Macklin, "Ethical Relativism in a Multicultural Society," *Kennedy Institute of Ethics Journal*, 8, 1 (1998): 1.

33. Barbara Herman, "Pluralism and the Community of Moral Judgment," in Heyd, *Toleration*, 62.

34. Horton cites Peter Nicholson's use of this distinction in Peter Nicholson, "Toleration as Moral Ideal," in *Aspects of Toleration: Philosophical Studies*, ed. John Horton and Susan Mendus (London: Methuen, 1985); see Horton, "Toleration as a Virtue," 30ff.

35. Leon R. Kass, "The Wisdom of Repugnance," *New Republic*, 216, 22 (June 2, 1997).

36. Ruth Macklin, *Against Relativism*, 51–52.

Chapter Four

On the Path to Presence

Sarah is an eighty-year-old woman who is a first generation American. She was raised in a traditional conservative Jewish home. Her husband died after 50 years of a strong marriage. She has three children. While her home is not kosher, she practices a variation of kosher-style eating, avoiding pork and not making dishes that combine meat and milk.

Two months ago, she was diagnosed with pancreatic cancer. Surgery was attempted, but the cancer was already in an advanced stage. Chemotherapy was started, but the cancer has progressed and is not responding to the medications. She is having difficulty eating because of the pressure of the tumor on the gastrointestinal track. Discussions are being held to determine whether or not treatments should be stopped and whether hospice care should be initiated. What must you anticipate in discussing with Sarah her wishes regarding the continuation of care?[1]

* * *

Mr. Harris, a sixty-eight-year-old black male, was scheduled to have his cancerous prostrate removed at a government hospital. Two days after scheduling the procedure, he called Karen, his nurse, in panic. He had spoken to several friends about his upcoming surgery, and now wanted to know about various forms of alternative treatments. Karen spent about an hour on the phone with him and gave him a great deal of information as well as phone numbers he could call to learn about other options. She realized that he was probably overwhelmed and frightened about his diagnosis.

Right before hanging up, Mr. Harris said, "You know I trust *you*, Karen; I just don't know if I trust the hospital to take care of me."[2]

* * *

Until we can acknowledge and seek to overcome these hurdles, cultural competency lies beyond our reach. The most significant, effective, and far-reaching path to address these obstacles lies in resuscitating the art of presence. While patient satisfaction no doubt involves medical efficacy and positive medical outcome, another vital though undervalued gem lies in health professionals' genuine, interpersonal, face-to-face encounter, that is, their presence with patients. Authentic rapport and caring on the part of physicians in particular play a major role, the key to which is imbedded in communication and presence.

Emmanuel Levinas' views of inter-human encounter and intersubjectivity offer a rich metaphysical base for positing and cultivating a virtue of presence in healthcare. Edith Wyschogrod describes Levinas' insights as an "ethical metaphysics" since he lays a conceptual foundation for highlighting the moral primacy of the other person.[3] The other person's presence to us naturally elicits and compels a response on our part, a response that is moral and one that affirms a mutual contract in which we are each ultimately responsible to the other. In my own response lies the fruition of my self, my personal being. This goes beyond the call to love my neighbor as myself. This demands that *loving my neighbor in itself constitutes myself*, as in "love thy neighbor as oneself."[4]

This fully contradicts the lamentably increasing social disposition in the U.S. and elsewhere of being-for-*oneself*. Levinas poses a metaphysical ground for presence that demands an authentic and committed being *for the other*, a being *towards* and *with* the other. When we apply this to the domain of cultural discourse, the Other represents no moral distance, but rather poses to me a moral duty, not in the sense of my gratuitously, generously acting from superficial obligation, but in my being naturally and inherently morally responsible for and to the Other. Therein lies my dignity, as here both erogatory and supererogatory coexist.

My moral responsibility to the Other is unavoidable. For Levinas, the other's presence, naturally expressed relationally, is embodied in the Other's *visage*, face. The Other's face literally acts as a perennial, embodied reminder of my accountability, not only to the Other whom I face here and now, but to all Others whose faces remain invisible, yet just as real and transparent. Encountering the face of one elicits desire and demand for equity and justice for all. My friend and respected physician and scholar John Balint implies as much in proposing that physicians' role not only encompasses duties to their individual patients but extends toward "addressing the socio-economic and psycho-social factors that impact health."[5]

Levinas' notion of *visage*, "face," is especially instructive in the context of discourse. The "face" we encounter is the "phenomenon that is the apparition of the Other" and this "epiphany of the face is visitation."[6] Thus the Other's presence makes itself evident naturally via a manifestation of the Other's face, a manifestation in which "the face speaks" to us originally through a "discourse." For Levinas, this encounter with the Other through the Other's face is our primal text: "The manifestation of the face is the first discourse. Speaking is first and foremost this way of coming from behind one's appearance, behind one's form; an opening in the opening."[7] In this way, the presence of the other's *visage*, or face, represents our original charge, "an irrefutable order—a commandment. . . . Consciousness is challenged [*mise en question*] by the face."[8] The Other's face obliges us to acknowledge, recognize, to respond, for "the face imposes on me and I cannot stay deaf to its appeal, or forget it . . . I cannot stop being responsible for its desolation. Consciousness loses its first place."[9] While this presence of the Other via face is a "summons to respond,"[10] I cannot help but respond in my own way, as *le Moi*, as who I am, as Ego.[11] This means that I remain "infinitely responsible in the face of the Other"[12] and thereby reconnect with what I naturally intuit of the Other. Moreover, this conveys a deeper sense of "person." As Abraham Heschel reminds physicians, "To heal a person, one must be a person."[13] Etymology offers a hint. *Persona*, *per-sona*, represents that through which comes sound. For this reason, the manifestation of compassion requires, as a necessary condition, presence.

This embodied encounter via the face is crucial to bear in mind given our cultural obsession with connecting technologies that preclude face-to-face encounter. For Levinas, the source of meaning lies in the face-to-face encounter, not one that is mediated through devices and screens. *Face-to-face rapport is itself a moral event*, one in which the patient, the Other, covertly embodies the request to be acknowledged, recognized, and responded to, a request to which the health professional or caregiver is morally called to heed. As genuine presence requires a face-to-face encounter, the intrinsically moral nature of communication becomes evident. Levinas distinguishes between the *saying* (*le dire*) and the *said* (*le Dit*). Saying constitutes a dynamic, unfolding communicative gesture as opposed to the static whatness of the said. In Levinas' terms, whereas "significance" refers to the content, what is said, or *le Dit*, "signification" refers to the saying itself, the expressiveness, *le Dire*, the relationality which is itself a moral domain. In the signification, the saying, lies the moral act.[14] To focus single-mindedly on the content, *le Dit*, detracts from the source of ethics, the saying itself, the communicative act or gesture, the embodied expression in a face-to-face encounter. Intersubjectivity is itself a moral event since the real significance of signification lies in the communicating.

The vital importance of face-to-face encounter should not be underestimated, again a critically relevant concern in a climate where information communication technologies (ICT) now play an all-pervasive role as *the* primary vehicle now communicating and where face-to-face communicating is becoming fast obsolete.[15] During a Communication, Medicine, and Ethics (COMET) symposium on views of meaningful presence and its application in the healthcare setting and relevance for healthcare communication, someone astutely raised a question as to whether presence can also be legitimately reconceived as "online presence," as, for instance, in the increasing use of online persona such as an anonymous "avatar."[16] In response, I offered my belief that genuine presence must be embodied.[17] In fact, the original meaning of avatar is thoroughly incarnational, from *avatāra* in the Bhagavadgita. Here the god Vishnu assumes human form as Krishna. Krishna is thus the incarnation of the divine in human form. It appears that the virtual now assumes a hegemony and even god-like status.[18] In any case, although interpersonal face-to-face exchange can misplace primacy on *le Dit* by reducing the interpersonal exchange to the "said," communication technologies, occurring as they do without embodied inter-presence, naturally shift from the "saying" to inevitably focus on content, *le Dit*.

Embodied presence takes on special meaning in Levinas' "ethical metaphysics." Our skin does not divide us from each other, but unites us, as with Maurice Merleau-Ponty's body-subject in interactive perception with the perceived world of experience, in which we are impressed upon and impress. As we are naturally embodied in the world, genuine meaning can only come about via our embodied existence. Furthermore, our embodiment consists in the evident truth that ours is a shared bodiliness. This shared bodiliness is implied in Julia Tao Lai Po-Wah's thesis that our biological and social heritage enables a shared universality.[19] While she posits the one-sidedness of patient-centered, physician-centered, and family-centered models, models that exacerbate cultural fault lines, she offers a way of integrating all three in her Confucian shared-decision model, respecting a patient's individual and relational, particularly familial, identity, and thus asserts common ground in relationality. Her affirmation in a sense reflects the deeper common ground of embodied co-presence. In view of embodied presence, emphasis upon embodiment and bodiliness itself plays a prominent role in familial relationality. Tao Lai reminds us of the moral imperative of filial piety and cites the Confucian classic *The Book of Filial Piety*, "The body, including our hair and skin, we receive from our parents. We dare not cause any injury to it, and this is the beginning of filial piety."[20] In this context of relational bodiliness, personal dignity and interpersonal dependency are not mutually exclusive, as they are often viewed as in our excessively individualized culture. As Tao

Lai asserts, "There is no question of loss of dignity for a Chinese elderly sick parent in being dependent on her children. She is fully entitled to this kind of dependency."[21]

In view of our shared bodiliness and embodied inter-presence, all sentient beings participate in its singular feature of temporariness, innate vulnerability, illness, and imperfection. Hence, the foremost Buddhist Noble Truth that suffering is universal. As in suffering, in Buddhist *dukkha*, in temporariness we all share in a fundamental dislocatedness. Indeed, Levinas' thinking here is somewhat akin to Buddhism. Our embodied presence beckons us to respond to others in order to alleviate others' suffering. This in turn liberates us from our self-imposed cocoon. The call of the other liberates us from self-concern and away from the centrifugal pull of our own individual being-toward-our-own-private-death that confines us within the dual prison of Space, only the local is real, and Time, only my own history matters. Rather, as Levinas would have it, the call of the other through the Other's *visage* and presence frees us to *be-for-others-in-a-future-beyond-my-death*.[22]

In this sense, presence as truly being *for* the other liberates me from my narrow spatiality (my world) and temporality (my history), and in our leap of faith into an undisclosed future, we do not live *for* the moment, but necessarily *in* the moment. For Levinas, the former is "base and vulgar."[23] The belief that only the now matters constitutes a moral lie, one which drives our current and future ecological predicament, a consequence of our ego-logical ground. Our inability to transcend this ground in order to allow for the "epiphany of the Other" is our contemporary failure.[24] This being for others in a future beyond my death clearly extends beyond Heiddegger's assertion of my individual being-towards-my-death. It also stretches further than Robert Jay Lifton's modes of my personal symbolic immortality which still remains self-oriented, representing my inability to accept *my* no-longer being. My being for others in a future beyond my death also calls for presence as a type of transcendence, a being-in-transcendence, and so freeing us (this is the demand of ethics) from the twofold prison of private Space and individual Time. Embodiment entails our openness to my and others' suffering and mortality. As Richard Cohen points out:

> Suffering and mortality, then, are first and foremost the suffering and mortality of the other, from whom one's own suffering, otherwise useless, takes on meaning. The significance of embodiment is neither attachment to self nor attachment to being but rather vulnerability to the other, hence, moral compassion.[25]

This vision towards a future without me, beyond my death, naturally broadens our notion of justice. Though Freud held that thinking of ourselves as not being is conceptually impossible, working towards a future beyond my death bears poignancy as a way to resist thinking in terms of inflated concerns of my individual rights and well-being. Embodied presence in this sense opens us to others' suffering and beckons our response, naturally a never-ending task, perpetually hindered when we confine ourselves to our own time-self dimension. Here, we touch upon the pulse of hope—to live *for* what is not yet by committing ourselves fully in the now, as in Camus' conviction that our best investment in the future is to give all to the present.

In summary, authentic presence demands being genuinely *there* with the patient, and this involves a being-with, being-for, being-in-relation, and being-in-transcendence. Being-*there* with a living, embodied person who happens to be a patient means encountering the patient's lived reality and not allowing my view, image, or concept of the patient from interfering with our encounter. Levinas says it better: "The face of the Other at each moment destroys and overflows the plastic image it leaves me, the idea existing to my own measure."[26] Being *with* and *for* the patient, sparked by the patient's *visage*, is a call for my response which is in itself a moral event. My primordial duty and fundamental commitment is to the other, an obligation for which I am accountable. My being *in relation* is in response to the Other's presence, which implicitly invites my responsiveness. And being *in transcendence* acknowledges that "In the face, the Other expresses his eminence, the dimension of height and divinity from which he descends."[27] Furthermore, this transcendence beckons that I am for the other beyond my own death, thus freeing me from my self-absorbed and self-imposed localized and historical prison.

It is only through embodied presence that we as caregivers can genuinely *give care*, *care for*, and empathize with the patient in her pain and suffering. Caring for another is fundamental. Nel Noddings emphasizes caring as life's most basic drive—a need to care-for and to be-cared-for. At its core, caring constitutes a moral disposition that Noddings asserts "involves stepping outside of one's personal frame of reference into the other's . . . we consider the other's point of view, his objective needs, and what he expects of us."[28] Along these lines, mutual embodied presence to each other represents a natural unfolding and reciprocity, an inter-presence, that encompasses both being impressed upon and impressing.

Recent neuroscientific research affirms the critical importance of bodiliness and inter-presence. Neuroscientist Marco Iacoboni finds that special brain cells called mirror neurons integrate what they "mirror" in ways that alter neuronal patterns that enable motor responses. For instance, they mirror gestures in ways that both imitate and coincide with what is seen, felt, or even imagined. Here there is evidence for a possible biological basis for empathy. As Iacoboni puts it, "mirror neurons fire when we see others ex-

pressing their emotions, as if we were making those facial expressions ourselves. By means of this firing, the neurons also send signals to emotional
brain centers in the limbic system to make us feel what other people feel."[29]

In his brilliant *Phenomenologie de la Perception*, Merleau-Ponty describes how illness thoroughly reminds us of our corporeal selves. Illness is
intensely personal, the experience of which has little to do with the abstract
template imposed upon that experience in the clinical encounter, and equating illness with that template betrays our philosophical conceit. The patient's
experience, his or her Ur-narrative, cannot be replaced by some systematic,
often reductionist conceptual schema. Levinas' "significance" cannot exist
apart from the access itself leading to it, the "signification." The communicating encompasses the journey toward meaning. This sheds a ray of light in
the case of clinical decision-making.

The signification of the decision to be made cannot be intelligible to
anyone but the person who had lived the past leading up to that decision.
Signification cannot be directly understood in a flash of light that illuminates
and chases the night from which it arises, that it unravels. It needs all the
density of the story.[30]

Our shared embodiment reminds us that our first duty is not inward, but
outward. The other's presence beckons us to respond to and work to relieve
and help heal the other's suffering. Healing is an endless labor, yet the aim
lies not in finishing but in confronting and struggling to embrace the task at
hand.

NOTES

1. Janice Selekman, "People of Jewish Heritage," in *Transcultural Health Care: A Culturally Competent Approach*, 2nd ed., ed. Larry D. Purnell and Betty J. Paulanka (Philadelphia:
F.A. Davis Company): 247.

2. Geri-Ann Galanti, *Caring for Patients from Different Cultures: Case Studies from
American Hospitals*, 2nd ed. (Philadelphia: University of Pennsylvania Press, 1997): 5.

3. Edith Wyschogrod, *Emmanuel Levinas: The Problem of Ethical Metaphysics*, 2nd ed.
(New York: Fordham University Press, 2000).

4. Cited in Levinas, *Humanism of the Other*, xxvii. How does this compare with Buddhism? On the surface, it appears to offend Buddhist ontology, falling back upon the self/other
distinction. Rather than asserting that, as in Buddhism, self *is* the neighbor or self *is* other, in
this case, self is *loving* other, neighbor.

5. John Balint, "Rethinking the Social Role of Physicians: The Importance of Physicians'
'Symbolic Acts,'" NYSBA *Health Law Journal*, 11, 3 (Summer/Fall 2006): 54. John Balint's
father, internationally renowned Hungarian psychotherapist and general physician Michael
Balint, is especially known for his classic and pioneering work on the physician-patient rela-
tionship and the therapeutic value of the physician, *The Doctor, the Patient, and the Illness*
(London: Tavistock Publications, 1957).

6. Levinas, *Humanism of the Other*, 31.

7. Levinas, *Humanism of the Other*, 31.

8. Levinas, *Humanism of the Other*, 32.

9. Levinas, *Humanism of the Other*, 32.

10. Levinas, *Humanism of the Other*, 32.

11. For Levinas, ego remains absolutely unique, in contrast to Buddhist *anatta*, no self, the truth of the absence of ego. Ego does not dissolve as the illusion it is in Buddhism. However, it dissolves its own self-absorption, its "dogmatic naivete in the face of the Other," *Humanism of the Other*, 36.

12. Levinas, *Humanism of the Other*, 35.

13. Abraham J. Heschel, *The Insecurity of Freedom* (New York: Noonday Press, 1966): 24–38.

14. This is a prevailing distinction in Emmanuel Levinas, *Otherwise than Being: Or Beyond Essence*, trans. Alphonso Lingis (Pittsburgh, PA: Duquesne University Press, 1981).

15. See Sherry Turkle, *Alone Together: Why We Expect More from Technology and Less from Each Other* (New York: Basic Books, 2011).

16. The title of our symposium was "Presence in Health Care Communication—Discursive and Ethical Dimensions," with Ulla Hellstrom Muhli, Jill Dales, José Carlos Gonçalves, Roxana Delbene, each offering insightful views on presence, June 29, 2011, Boston.

17. I raised this issue of avatar presence during our college's President's Day semi-annual session, the topic centering on Technology and the Teaching/Learning Process, Jan. 13, 2011.

18. Moral matters are profound. When our anonymous virtual personae rise above the boundaries of bodiliness, this inevitably impacts upon online and offline codes of behavior, socialization, and civility.

19. Julia Tao Lai Po-Wah, "A Confucian Approach to a 'Shared Family Decision Model' in Health Care: Reflections on Moral Pluralism," in Englehardt, *Global Bioethics*, 154–79.

20. Tao Lai, 164.

21. Tao Lai, 164.

22. Levinas, *Humanism of the Other*, 27ff.

23. Levinas, *Humanism of the Other*, 28.

24. Levinas, *Humanism of the Other*, 28.

25. Richard Cohen, Introduction to Levinas' *Humanism of the Other*, xxxiii.

26. Emmanuel Levinas, *Totality and Infinity*, trans. Alphonso Lingis (Pittsburgh, PA: Duquesne University Press, 1969, 1961): 51.

27. Levinas, *Totality and Infinity*, 262. For further discussion of presence in the context of Buddhist teachings, see Michael C. Brannigan, "Presence in Suffering: Lessons from the Buddhist Four Noble Truths," *Eubios Journal of Asian and International Bioethics*, 20 (November 2010): 173–79.

28. Nel Noddings, *Caring: A Feminine Approach to Ethics and Moral Education*, 2nd ed. (Berkeley: University of California Press, 1984), 24.

29. Marco Iacoboni, *Mirroring People: The Science of Empathy and How We Connect with Others* (New York: Picador/Farrar, Straus and Giroux): 119.

30. Levinas, *Humanism of the Other*, 20.

Chapter Five

Cultivating Presence When
There Is Distrust

Mr. Ahmed recently moved to the U.S. from Egypt to join his family. Having symptoms of Hodgkin's disease, he was admitted for treatment and assessment for chemotherapy. Neither he nor his family was conversant in English.

He and his family were deeply offended by the staff's efforts to inquire into his health history and offered no response to many of the nurses' questions, which he regarded as rude and intrusive. And when the staff insisted on his signature for written consent, they were met with resistance and distrust.

At one point while sipping soup, he choked and required a tracheostomy tube. Inserting the tube was quite difficult and resulted in anoxic encephalopathy. With severe loss of oxygen to his brain, and remaining in a coma, though not brain dead, his situation deteriorated.

His family was extremely offended when the medical staff approached them to discuss treatment options including forgoing treatment. The family remained deeply suspicious of the staff's motives.[1]

* * *

Before we move on to offer more practical strategies to help cultivate this genuine sense of presence in the clinical setting, we need to tackle the thorny systemic matter of authority and, more specifically, how we tend to assign trust in that authority. In the following, consider first the question of authority and trust in the healthcare institution, after which we examine the related issue of the authority we often grant to media narrative and images.

TRUSTING THE INSTITUTION

Ensuring efficacy in cultural competency work encounters the more discreet problematic of assessing internal mechanisms that aim to measure levels of cultural competency. These internal performance mechanisms respond to an institutional need to not only cultivate an environment that is culturally as well as morally sensitive and thus be publicly perceived to be trustworthy of such, but also to monitor procedures and outcomes. How can we generate public trust in an institution that is part of a wider healthcare system which is often perceived as essentially self-serving and untrustworthy? This is of course where institutional structures are in place to oversee and monitor.

However, institutional measures, though necessary, are not in themselves sufficient enough to warrant public trust in the institution. As Onora O'Neill tellingly underscores, an institutional entity that has developed strategies to enhance its trustworthiness (for example through ethics committees, ethics officers and consultants, compliance departments) is not necessarily one which at the same time generates public trust.[2] What enables trustworthiness does not necessarily bring about the "placing of trust," or trusting. Her analyses of recent healthcare organizational hurdles in the U.K. illustrate this and can be applied to cultural competency mechanisms. For instance, the process of systemic internal monitoring by way of audit mechanisms can be counterproductive to its aim. In the U.S., the 1999 Texas Advance Directives Act may have culled further institutional traction in an effort to improve the state's healthcare institutions' trustworthiness regarding the plaguing issues of withdrawing medically "futile" treatment, but they have not guaranteed public trust in these same institutions. Within the Act's guidelines for resolving disputes we read:

1. The physician's refusal to comply with the patient's or surrogate's request for treatment must be reviewed by a *hospital-appointed medical or ethics committee* in which the attending physician does not participate. . . .
4. If the ethics-consultation process fails to *resolve* the dispute, the hospital, working with the family, must make reasonable efforts to transfer the patient's care to another physician or institution willing to provide the treatment requested by the family. . . .
6. The patient or surrogate may request a court-ordered time extension, which should be granted only if the judge determines that there is a *reasonable likelihood of finding a willing provider of the disputed treatment*."[3] [author italics]

Upon close reading of these stipulations, "resolution" appears to be a default position in favor of professionals in the institution who urge withdrawing futile treatment, even in the face of family opposition. More generally, even though healthcare policy and guideline documents are in principle grounded upon moral theory and designed for morally sound application within institutions, to what degree is this actualized in practice? Are such policies more reflective of unfair institutional bias? Along these lines, internal auditing mechanisms help to create a bureaucracy and formal distancing which by themselves become objects of distrust. Evidence-based emphases illustrate this "audit culture" in healthcare. Yet can we sufficiently measure "cultural competence" in similar ways?

No doubt, monitoring and measuring cultural competency has its benefits. Institutions can feel more secure in having clear objectives, procedures to meet these objectives, and a scale to assess outcomes. (To review some of these thoughtful and no doubt helpful assessment models see the note below.)[4] These can enhance institutional accountability and rate high grades in accreditation schemas. Yet monitoring performance through some institutional lens can also further intensify an internal "divide" whereby those on the "inside," physicians, nurses, etc., on the front lines working with patients from diverse backgrounds, now held accountable, can feel as intrusive. As a start, who establishes the appropriate procedures and by what standards? In achieving cultural competency, if the assessment of "outcomes based" rests upon "following prescribed procedures" in the way of so-called "best practices" or "evidence-based" application, what does this mean? Who prescribes the prescription? Experts? Administrators? Ethicists? And why would procedural efficacy be a sufficient enough condition for legitimacy? As O'Neill asserts:

> In effect, those who are audited are held accountable not only for achieving *outcomes* and *standards*, or alternatively for following *prescribed procedures*, but *for achieving outcomes and standards by following prescribed procedures*. Managerial and bureaucratic disciplines are to be combined in a belt-and-braces approach to securing trustworthiness. Unfortunately, the prescribed procedures sometimes obstruct rather than contribute to the outcomes and standards demanded, and sometimes distort the priorities, the aims and the efficiency of the institutions and professions to which they are applied.[5]

While important to bear in mind O'Neill's operative terms "sometimes obstruct" and "sometimes distorts," this sort of 'compliance ethics' is not a substitute for thorough moral analysis. However, I've seen such compliance approach to ethics in many settings, the skewed minimalist belief that acting ethically amounts to acting within institutional and legal parameters. To illustrate, although the membership on hospital ethics committees should include a legal professional versed in healthcare ethics (and should *not* include that institution's own legal counsel), the violation of such rule is not uncommon, particularly for committee members used to a cultural and institutional ethos that associates moral justification with legal permissibility. That legal voice can also be the overpowering and overriding factor in cases of moral conflict presented to the committee. Knowing legal boundaries is crucial, but not in itself determinative. Along similar lines, the voice of the putative "ethicist" can be wrong-headedly conceived to be representative of moral authority, a perversion of the proper role of the "ethicist" in helping to guide the group to some reasonable recommendation, a recommendation that only makes sense when various parties and stake-holders' perspectives are acknowledged and weighed through reasoned consensus, which, by the way, is another sticking point in committee decision-making—what constitutes reasoned consensus and what value do we assign it? When performance standards for cultural competency become formal, official, and transparent, bureaucratizing an inherently complex process stands in danger of betraying the fundamental aim of cultivating public trust, a betrayal that emerges when literal adherence to procedures overrides the spirit behind the procedures so that measurement of cultural competency is transformed into a strictly quantitative matter.[6]

Narrative and Image

Why do we still often uncritically defer to an institution's internal mechanism of monitoring and safeguarding? Why do we capriciously trust an untrustworthy or unreliable system? This all-too-common uncritical posture reflects in some ways our trust in the authority we excessively attribute to media narratives. Anecdotes and stories are a driving force in U.S. bioethics as media accounts particularly through major outlets such as CNN, MSNBC, Fox News, *Time*, and *Newsweek* are particularly powerful. With its consummate power to convince us and themselves they represent the voice of the public, media have become, as George Walden calls them, the "new elite."[7] Particularly when it comes to public expectations of healthcare and new medical "breakthroughs," media's power, too long neglected in U.S. bioethics, assumes unquestioned authority in shaping public impressions, fears, and hopes. Abrogating its mission to inform in balanced fashion, media is instead more inclined to stoke the flames of controversy via narratives.

Yet, as seduction requires both the seducer and the participation of the seduced, in our uncritical embrace of media accounts, we willingly comply in our seduction, and therein, for all its dramatic flair, lies the peril of narrative. It can lead, distort, exaggerate, deceive, and detract from real issues and their genuine complexity that requires thoughtful, reasoned, deliberation. Peering as voyeurs into the human spectacle of identifiable sufferers and victims serves to distract, and what more alluring spectacle is there than that of others' suffering? Exposing stories trumps careful consideration of questions these stories unearth, questions that demand the utmost in digging beneath the surface.

What especially breathes life into the narrative, especially now in our screen-centric culture, is the image, especially the image of another's pain and suffering. We tend to trust that these images capture truth. Yet images of others' suffering pose painful questions particularly when we self-critically reflect on *what it means to view the images*. Recall photojournalist Kevin Carter's riveting photo, shot during Sudan's terrible famine, that appeared in the March 26, 1993, *New York Times* of a small Sudanese girl, stooped over on the barren soil, barely able to crawl, dying from hunger and helplessness, while a vulture lurks and waits in the background. Carter's photo earned him a Pulitzer Prize. A year after the award, the thirty-three-year-old Carter committed suicide. He once confessed to a friend, "I'm really, really sorry I didn't pick the child up." How do we deal with the agonizing memory of others' suffering? The spectacle of others' misery, whether in a photo or in the packaged blur of moving images from CNN, MSNBC, Fox News, ABC, etc., may captivate us in all-consuming ways, particularly under the crushing moral weight of the question 'How to Respond?' What does it mean for us to observe these images of others' suffering? What is it about the image that we trust? What kind of knowledge do images convey? How much can we digest? Do they inform us? Transform us?

In the context of intercultural awareness, an implicit trust in the image is all the more troubling given the image's fundamental paradox. They appear to convey a sense of reality as it is, so that in a sense we all see the same thing, like the stunned faces of Haitians huddling together by the rubble of what was once Port-au-Prince, like African children dying from malaria that can be treated through proper antenatal malarial infection and insecticide-treated nets (somewhere in the world, most likely Africa, a child dies every thirty seconds from malaria), and like malnourished Americans in Appalachia. At the same time, each image is not only shot from the photographer's reference point, but each one of us also views the same image through our own reference point, our own lens of perception and imagination. We therefore *do not all see the same thing* as our interpretations vary. There is no "we" that views the same photo. As Susan Sontag deftly points out, "No 'we' should be taken for granted when the subject is looking at other people's pain."[8]

None of this undermines the immense value of the image. We need the image. Images spark us to ask questions. Whether we can more properly situate the image within its political and historical context, however, is another matter. It is all too easy to simply allow the image to be everything we know, as in our 'knowledge of a book' through the movie. Images, moreover, have a way of assaulting our sympathies so that, although we may feel helpless, we also feel compelled to act. If there is any moral core to sympathy, it lies in transforming the sympathizer into acting. In this way, images can be an invaluable vehicle to demonstrate our connectedness with one another. Images also keep memory alive and for many of us, like forgotten elderly, may be our only connection to the past.

At the same time, again in the interest of intercultural awareness, we abuse images when we insensitively violate others' privacy and dignity in the name of the public interest and right to be informed. Consider the images of bloated bodies just after the Jonestown mass "suicide" in Guyana, or the online footage of Daniel Pearl's brutal slaughter. Media representation via images can breach the dignity of both the living and the dead, as in CNN's televised account in the aftermath of Haiti's devastating earthquake of Anderson Cooper sticking a microphone under thick rubble so that we become privy to the screams of a daughter while her family desperately tries to lift the debris.

While we often trust the image to convey the entire story, the truth, the image is only a shot in time, freezing a particular moment, a moment which is merely a fragment of a broader context. That moment in time is in reality a fusion of historic, economic, social, and cultural forces, discovery of which only comes with extended reflection and study. Until then, we remain spectators of an antiseptic construction of what is real. What is left out of the image is just as real, if not more so.

CULTIVATING CLINICAL PRESENCE

How does all this relate to our interpersonal, clinical encounter with the patient? There exists a disturbing parallel between how we view the image and how we view the patient. Our first impression of the patient typically comes from the initial medical interview and clinical assessment, a domain in which physician presence, in the full sense of attentiveness and listening as described earlier, is crucial. Otherwise, like the image, we mistakenly believe that the impression conveys the patient's story, the patient's truth.

As a starting point, how does the patient present his or her complaint? Here, physician presence comes to the fore, and this involves acknowledging that how a patient presents his or her complaint may well be culturally inscribed. For instance, Asian patients often resort to bodily metaphors to describe their perceptions of their ailment. A Chinese patient may describe her symptoms in terms of a "fire in the chest" or an "injured heart." A Korean patient may allude to his "body fire."[9] Regardless of metaphors, it is critical that we not focus *solely* on the complaint. A somatic complaint regarding tiredness, headaches, or pain may mask other issues. A psychological complaint such as depression or sadness is generally a prelude to further concerns.

Culture understandably imprints ways in which we present our complaints. Communicative assumptions in Western cultures are not necessarily shared by others.[10] Muslim patients who appear more silent and reticent may on that account seem less communicative and open. Yet we display a cultural bias in presuming that authentic communication necessarily entails openness, directness, clarity, and overt verbal self-expression, a bias that comes to the surface in the course of the medical interview and a primary focus on the patient's complaint. Cultural competency clearly requires that we be aware of these communicative biases, biases that color the level of engagement and discourse.

The healthcare professional's presence to the patient also involves recognizing patients' different educational levels, all the more reason to avoid homogenizing cultural viewpoints. While Internet access is now more commonplace, it is clearly dangerous to wrongly assume a patient's knowledge base on the basis of some presumed universal access to Internet information.[11] To illustrate, in an effort to construct some reasonable set of recommendations for guidelines regarding hospital policies throughout the Kansas City region to address medical futility, there was an urgent need to meet with vulnerable groups, particularly Latinos, who represent a significant proportion of the population in the area. Our focus group discussions needed to start from the basics and discuss the more fundamental issues of patients' rights to be properly informed in order to make an educated degree of consent. Studies have indicated that Latino women are especially prone to risk from cancer due to unequal educational and healthcare access.[12]

A plaguing issue in the physician-patient encounter lies in the matter of time. Under the tyranny of time-pressure, establishing and building rapport with patients through presence seems naïve. Can we ascertain the patient's true concerns, the patient's truth, with the little time we have to genuinely *be* with the patient? Cultivating trust and rapport requires quality time, and this involves a socializing through "small talk."[13] In view of patient vulnerability due to health, education, social status, ethnicity, age, gender, and so on, establishing rapport requires small steps to build trust. The skill lies in balancing small talk with more serious talk about details, the medical facts, and this in turn requires that we patiently avoid rushing headlong into strictly medical matters.

Listening, more than talk, is the key to engagement, listening that is not simply hearing what is said but, as Theodore Reik reminds us, "listening with the third ear." As in climbing a slope, the engagement is a gradual inquiry from 'easy' issues like pain, sleep habits, and appetite to the more complex and delicate concerns like body image, bodily decline, sexual dysfunction, and mortality. As a result of presence, this engagement further helps to ensure patient trust.

What is the patient's truth? The truth of the encounter? Certainly not some objective, static, reified entity. The encounter quite starkly illustrates shifting contexts of truth(s), and that truths regarding the patient transcend mere history taking and fact finding. One must often go beyond the situation's immediacy to discover its truth. Tseng and Streltzer offer an example of a Filipino-American male patient who deliberately lies to his physician regarding compliance with medication, and does so out of respect for the physician's authority and to not display disharmony and opposition to the physician, a trait apparently reinforced in his cultural upbringing. "After the initial visit, the patient's blood pressure was found to be 160/104, so the physician prescribed an antihypertensive medicine for him. At the follow-up visit, the patient's blood pressure was still high: 162/98." Upon questioning, the patient repeatedly told the physician that he was taking the medication. The physician then spoke with the patient's wife, who was there for each visit but was silent, who then informed the physician that her husband stopped taking the medication after the first dose because of dizziness. According to his wife, her husband "dared not to tell the doctor that he did not like the medicine prescribed for him, and thus kept saying 'Yes, doctor!' obediently. . . . This illustrates how the patient is relating to the physician and responding to the physician's inquiry by deferring to authority (with respect and no opposition), as he was raised to do in his culture."[14]

This matter of the patient's 'truth' in intercultural settings naturally includes the translational fabric of interpretation and the role of interpreters. The translator comes as close as possible to the literal meaning of *what is expressed*. The interpreter, on the other hand, assumes the more comprehensive role of a synthetic, contextual hermeneutic of translating in a way that approximates the *spirit behind what is expressed*, considering contextual nuances and the like. Whereas translation is formulaic, interpretation is more contextual. A good translator need not be a good interpreter. A sound interpreter, particularly in matters of intercultural health, must be especially knowledgeable of and sensitive to specific cultures as well as being a solid translator. When engaged with a patient who knows little or no English, who then is the appropriate interpreter? Consider the case of Mrs. Chen.

Mrs. Chen is an eighty-four-year-old Chinese woman who speaks very little English. She has metastatic cancer, and her prognosis is quite grim. She lives with her son, and he has always served as her translator. According to accounts from the healthcare team, Mrs. Chen knows that she has cancer and that her time is limited. Her physician explained that he told her himself, using Mrs. Chen's son to translate:

> One day a nurse is in the room and mentions something about the cancer diagnosis. Mrs. Chen is clearly shocked and sinks into a deep depression. When he arrives later that day, her son is outraged that the nurse would tell his

mother about the cancer diagnosis. . . . Mrs. Chen's son had not been translating exactly what the doctor said . . . he never told her that she had cancer. He saw his role as protector of his mother and thought that if he told her the truth about her condition, he would devastate her and remove all hope and possibility of enjoyment during her last days and months. [15]

Given an inherent problematic regarding the use of family members as interpreters due precisely to their proximity to the patient, this paradox of proximity consists of the difficulty in formulating a clear enough picture of the circumstance due to closeness, and issues tend to become increasingly intense when concerns are all the more volatile such as one's quality of living towards the end of life.

In an intercultural healthcare setting, the most volatile issues concern matters of the body and bodily privacy, children's care, matters related to pregnancy and birth, cancer, sexual orientation, menstruation and menopause, and death. Consider the sensitive issue of bodily privacy and intrusion. The physical exam as we customarily think of it is not a universal feature in medical examination and bodily inspection is not accepted by all cultures. Direct bodily intrusions such as prostate exams can therefore present a problem for patients who either do not understand the procedure, perhaps from not having the procedure and its rationale clearly explained in comprehensible language, or who resist bodily probes we as a society 'tolerate.' Even without physical contact, the mere act of revealing certain parts of the body may cause discomfort. Many Muslim women prefer to wear the veil even during physical examinations.

What is at issue is not simply the matter of bodiliness but the association of bodiliness with identity, self. Our bodiliness is a conduit for thinking about personal identity and self. [16] Clearly, the cascade of exams and diagnostic procedures and tests such as MRIs, drawing blood, pelvic exams, and spinal taps adds further reason to be fully aware of and sensitive to views of bodiliness and self-construal among all patients, not just those from other cultures. Claustrophobia crosses cultures, and assigning an MRI can have devastating effects on certain patients. Furthermore, this body-self link generates issues at cross-purposes with the aim of medical exams, as in the case of Mexican parents who requested that a gynecologist exam their sixteen-year-old daughter in order to verify her virginity, as virginity is desired prior to marriage. [17] Though perhaps culturally compelling (as explanation), their reasoning is clearly at odds with medical teleology (as justification). Does cultural competence and sensitivity require that the physician accommodate their request? Is there a way to accommodate without violating the aim of the medical exam?

Clinical Strategies

Active Listening

The medical interview offers us the opportunity to cultivate presence from the start. Here especially, active listening is the building block for presence, an active listening that engages the whole person.[18] We communicate our messages in three fundamental ways: what we say, how we say it (body language, speech tonality, pitch, and rhythm), and what we do not say. All three ways intertwine with each other. In a Missouri hospital, the ethics officer, also a good friend, shared with me concerns that patients had informed him of their difficulty comprehending what an Indian physician was telling them on account of the physician's rapid speech. Pace affects the message. Language barriers constitute one of the biggest obstacles in communicating with Chinese patients, illustrating all the more the imperative of active listening. With Chinese patients, it is especially important to avoid phrasing medical matters in negative ways and, instead, ask positive-oriented questions.[19] Respecting space and avoiding direct eye contact is also critical. And although sitting next to each other is often the preferred mode of discourse, it is important that the physician maintain some level of formality, for instance by using family names instead of the more informal ones we tend to take for granted. Also, bear in mind that Chinese women tend to keep their family names, even after marriage.

While we ordinarily attribute more importance to what we actually say, the words we use, our overt verbal narrative, studies reveal that we actually ascribe more meaning to both how we speak and what is not spoken, delivered through bodily cues. Clinical oncology consultant Elisabeth Macdonald reveals patient attentiveness at 60% for nonverbal cues, 35% for tone of voice, and 5% to the spoken words.[20] Bodily presence therefore remains a crucial component in interpersonal communication. This is important to keep in mind as we increasingly communicate with each other digitally. Our sociocultural love affair with communication information technologies may better enable connecting from a distance. Our attachment to these devices at the same time disables personal, face-to-face interconnectedness, so that we are becoming disembodied beings.[21] Yet because active listening requires that we listen to both what is not said as well as what is said, meaning only comes about through our bodily being in the world.

Active listening requires that we learn the most difficult language of all, the language of silence. As Swiss philosopher Max Picard reminds us, silence is the ground of speech, without which speech is meaningless.[22] Active listening is deliberately attentive to silence in the clinical setting where patients experience vulnerability and intimate suffering. In such a setting, listening to the patient's silence requires that we avoid the temptation to control the communicative agenda through speech and jargon that in effect suppresses the deeper truths that only silence can reveal. As the Bengali poet and Nobel Prize winner Rabindranath Tagore writes, "The small truth has words that are clear; the great truth has great silence." Discovering the patient's "truth" through attentiveness to a patient's silence is increasingly complicated in a culture that thrives on what is spoken, what is expressly said. Presence in the sense of being for and with the other allows silence to have a 'say' in our conversation with the patient.

Pace

The patient occupies an inherently vulnerable position on levels of health condition, income, social status, education, race, ethnicity, gender, and age, among others. Nonetheless, the patient must be the moral center of concern in medicine. This means that we address the physician-patient power imbalance through empowering the patient to have a vital voice in setting the pace of the encounter and medical interview. For instance, when we communicate with Native-Americans, as with other groups, it is disrespectful to speak loudly and quickly, as I believe it is in general. It is also bad-mannered to name those who have died, one reason why kinship terms among Native Americans, for example "maternal grandfather," are preferable. And because Native Americans generally avoid complaining about pain unless it is within the intimate circle of family and close friends, the physician must allow the patient to set the pace. Surely the physician needs to have a plan, pursue that plan, and provide direction and guidance for the patient for the benefit of the patient. However, managing the agenda in this way is distinct from controlling it. The physician's management style can command the encounter in subtle ways such as interruptions and closed questions that preclude the patient from revealing more of the patient's truth, the all-important context behind the initial complaint. Another strategy to control the agenda lies in focusing solely upon the presenting complaint. In this way, the complaint becomes *the problem*, apart from the broader context of the patient's personal, familial, and social history and habits. Presence requires that we bracket, as in the phenomenological sense of bracketing or *epoche*, our own agenda in order to be genuinely present to, for, and with the other. In this way, we fully listen to the patient's story and not our own.

No doubt, medical tests are critical in order to establish proper diagnoses, especially in view of medical uncertainties. Despite popular views and expectations, medicine remains an inexact science as each patient is unique and responds to health conditions and treatments in distinctive ways. In the face of this uncertainty, medical techniques, diagnostic procedures, and tests offer some measure of assurance. At the same time, when reliance on these techniques and procedures *displaces* interpersonal engagement and inter-presence with the patient, the center of concern switches from the person of the patient to treatment modalities. Treatment measures trump the person being treated. In Akira Kurasawa's classic film *Ikiru* (To Live), one pivotal scene depicts patient Kenji Watanabe's physicians who appear fixed on the x-ray image of Watanabe's malignant stomach tumor. There is shelter in addressing the image, at arms length from the patient. Treating the patient who is suffering is much more confounding, unsettling, and demanding. Watanabe's suffering is profoundly and indelibly real. Yet when images *replace* the patient in the hierarchy of importance, becoming more real than the reality they depict, we enter the wasteland of what Jean Baudrillard terms the "hyperreal," when image, simulation, and technique are not only just as real as the real, but in effect are more "real." All this undercuts the healing power of presence with its implicit faith in what we can learn from our encounter with the patient. Instead, we place our faith in technique.

Reciprocity

Pratityasamutpada, or codependent origination, one of the most profound Buddhist teachings, signifies a fundamental, inescapable, and synergistic interconnectedness among all living beings so that every act constitutes both cause and effect. When applied to the noble profession of medicine, it reinforces the conviction that relieving suffering can only unfold in a climate of trust. I use "noble" deliberately since medicine ultimately intends to address and relieve suffering, and what more noble purpose is there? Without trust, a situation that potentially leads to healing transforms into one of doubt and suspicion. Reciprocity comes into play since genuine presence on the health professional's part naturally beckons response from patient and family, an inter-presence, hence the reciprocating nature of presence. And this reciprocity helps cultivate and sustain an indispensable trust for healing. The medical team's genuine and felt presence conveys to the patient the thoroughly profound communiqué to the patient that he or she is ultimately valued as a person and will be cared for in the best way they can. This message naturally, though not always, evokes the patient's favorable response.

CONCLUDING REMARKS

Active listening, pace, and reciprocity are basic strategies that help to nurture presence in the sense of truly being present to, for, and with the patient. The physician as healer is a professional who, in the desire to heal, offers her expertise, experience, and competence *to* the patient. The physician as healer is a professional who is also "present-*for*" the patient in that his or her commitment to the patient's well-being rests upon a humane convenantal relationship with the patient, an implicit pact that goes deeper that one which is contractual and minimalist. The physician as healer is a professional who is also "present-*with*" the patient, in partnership and working together with patient, surrogate, and family to promote the patient's well-being and uphold the patient at the center of moral concern. And, as described earlier, the physician as healer is a professional who is "present-in-*transcendence*." The deep mystery of the physician-patient interpersonal encounter transcends immanence. Here, reason and science meet their limits as faith and trust occupy a privileged place in the interpersonal encounter, one that is at the same time sacred.

Cultivating these ingredients of presence—active listening, pace, and reciprocity—remains enormously difficult within our U.S. healthcare system. Because our healthcare system tends to represent deep-rooted cultural values, the health professional's predicament is one that is in turn sociocultural. Our most palpable sociocultural quandary lies in our addiction to quick time, to speed. [23] Despite numerous time-saving technologies, we have less time to save, are busier than ever. In what Alan Lightman calls our "wired world" we work at a more frantic pace, faster and longer, without slowing down, a nervous society, on edge, unable to stop. [24] Ensconced in never-ending multitasks and projects that consume our attention, under the weight of deadlines, we've sliced up our hours into efficient units of time, with no time to waste, to pause, reflect, to simply not have to think about what one needs to think about nor time for inner quiet to imagine. In the process we have atrophied movement as we jump from one moment to the next. As we see in healthcare communication, though communication is a dialectic of words, expression, and silence, we atrophy communication when we focus only on the spoken words.

This is more than a matter of pondering time's mystery. Actually, its essence, if we can call it that, lies in *how we live time*. There is an important distinction between what time is and what we think of it. We mistakenly believe that time *is* how we think of it, and this naturally affects how we think of everything else, ourselves, others, our experiences, our lives, and our worldviews. Under this misconception, we lose sense of continuous, coherent time, time as duration. [25] Deluded, we slice time up into moments and think of time as fragmentary, without a center, an aim, without *telos* or overarching sense of purposeful living. At high speed, we stand still.

All this affects our moral behavior since how we view time shapes how we view our world, ourselves, the other, and what it means to interact with the other. Fragmenting time into moments naturally affects how we act within those moments. Whereas moral reasoning demands that we acknowledge a situation's complexity and, in turn, time's duration, living in the momentary dissolves this so that in the rush we find no time to pause to reflect on consequences of our actions.

Consumed by an incessant need to accomplish as much as we can in less time, we never have enough time to do it all as we run from deadline to deadline. Social anthropologist Thomas Erikson explains this via the formula: the more data ("information glut") we squeeze into time, the less time there is to filter the data, so that we feel overwhelmed by time. [26] Communication information technologies enable us to stay "connected" and we find ourselves ensnared in a range of diverse directions through which we multitask. Yet our ability to stay singularly focused on one task at a time is growing obsolete. In similar fashion, medicine moves forward in multiple contexts, appearing increasingly disjointed and without a coordinating center. Fragmentation in our health system threatens continuity and quality of patient care.

Under this tyranny of Time in which the patient's problem, the patient's truth, is more likely to be understood solely within diagnostic categories that objectify the patient's subjective experience of illness, and the patient's complaint is through default translated as *the* problem, how can health professionals *embody* presence with their patients? Under the constraints of time, efficiency rules the day as we attempt to address the complaint and resolve it. In the complex labyrinth of our health systems, providers face institutional pressures to perform cost effectively and thereby risk shifting the patient away from medicine's moral center. Under the axe of time, genuine presence, being where-we-are-and-with-whom-we-are, evaporates. Rather than actively listen to what is said, how it is said, and what is left unsaid, we listen more to our agenda and, in the process, pull ourselves away from the patient with and to whom we are present. Fixed to our own narrative of the patient, we commit the error about which the Buddhist Nagarajuna warned us in his *Mulamadhyamikakarika*—instead of seeing what is real, we redefine the real as ideas and concepts—the patient is now a condition. In doing so, we find comfort in a familiar biomedical zone detached from the patient's reality. At the same time, in our interpersonal encounter's moral event, we relinquish our moral commitment to be present with one who suffers.

In my work with patients, particularly hospice patients, my most meaningful lessons have come from those who were dying and knew they were dying. These patients have taught me that in their vulnerability they are also remarkably intuitive. They especially have a way of sensing others' authenticity and whether or not these others—physicians, nurses, hospital staff, family, friends, and so on—are genuinely *there-with-them*. I suspect that when we ourselves are in similar circumstances of vulnerability, we can intuit the attitude and disposition of our caregiver and sense whether or not he or she *cares for* us or simply *attends to* us. To the patient, we health professionals and caregivers also represent power. The patient hears not only what we say but what we choose not to say. Our bodies cannot help but give it away: our eyes, where we look, what we do with our hands, whether we seem fidgety, nervous, comfortable, or confident, how often we glance at our watch, whether we've turned off our pagers, whether and where we stand or sit, whether we write more or listen more, and most importantly whether we are sincere. Though non-quantifiable, sincerity emits these clues. Our physical environment also gives it away. Do we meet in a private setting? Is it quiet? Do tables, desks, chairs, computers, laptops, notes, clipboards, and other physical barriers separate us from the patient, to whom these barriers represent walls of authority and inaccessibility?

Cultivating the virtue of presence particularly in the context of intercultural awareness and sensitivity faces the enormous challenges discussed above. And time is of the essence in that it is not about how much time we have, but how we live it. Presence is ultimately a matter of practicing and fostering the art of using the little time we have, which may be all the time we really need, in the best way we can. Along with experience and expertise, we need to infuse competency with presence, and how we embody our presence with our patient ultimately makes all the difference. *How we are with the patient*, the person before us, constitutes the nobility of who we are as humans.

NOTES

1. A.I. Meleis and A. Jonsen, "Ethical Crises and Cultural Differences," *Western Journal of Medicine* 138, no. 6, June 1983: 889–892; in M. Brannigan and J. Boss, *Healthcare Ethics in a Diverse Society* (New York: McGraw-Hill, 2001), 486–87.

2. Onora O'Neill, *Autonomy and Trust in Bioethics* (Cambridge: Cambridge University Press, 2002): 118ff.

3. Robert D. Truog, "Tackling Medical Futility in Texas," *The New England Journal of Medicine* 357, 1 (July 5 2007); see full text of law at http://tlo2.tlc.state.tx.us/statutes/docs/HS/content/htm/hs.002.00.000166.00.htm).

4. Cultural competency assessment models include: Minnesota Department of Human Services, *Guidelines for Culturally Competent Organizations*, 2nd ed., May 2004, at http://www.leg.state.mn.us/docs/2005/other/050050.pdf; National Center for Cultural Competence, Georgetown University Child Development Center, at http://www.georgetown.edu/research/gucdc/nccc/ncccorgselfassess.pdf; J.R. Betancourt, A.R. Green, and J.E. Carrillo, *Cultural Competence in Health Care: Emerging Frameworks and Practical Approaches* (New York: The Commonwealth Fund; 2002); D. Andrulis, T. Delbianco, L. Avakian, and Y. Shaw-Taylor, *Conducting a Cultural Competence Self-Assessment*, at http://www.consumerstar.org/pubs/Culturalcompselfassess.pdf; Lumetra, *The Cultural Competence Self-Assessment Protocol for Managed Care Organizations*; *Developing a Self-Assessment Tool for Culturally and Linguistically Appropriate Services in Local Public Health Agencies: Final Report* (Rockville, MD: U.S. DHHS; 2003).

5. O'Neill, *Autonomy and Trust*, 132.

6. We see this in higher education where individual departments and their faculty are pressured to achieve outcomes most often in terms of enrollment numbers and majors. There is a lack of parity in establishing and measuring criteria for "success." Faculty in general, humanities and arts faculty in particular, do not historically tend to measure success in their fields via head counts, numbers of majors, class enrollments, and retention rates. Have internal account-

ability and measurability standards eroded further trust in educational quality? Can there be authentic trust in an academic institution that faces pressure from all sides to survive as well as thrive?

7. George Walden, *The New Elites: Making a Career in the Masses* (London: Allen Lane, Penguin Press, 2000).

8. Susan Sontag, *Regarding the Pain of Others* (New York: Picador/Farrar, Straus and Giroux, 2003): 7.

9. Tseng and Streltzer, *Cultural Competence in Health Care*, 27.

10. See the instructive account of Min-Sun Kim, *Non-Western Perspectives on Human Communication: Implications for Theory and Practice* (Thousand Oaks, CA: Sage Publications, 2002).

11. Betty Chang et al., "Bridging the Digital Divide: Reaching Vulnerable Populations," *Journal of the American Medical Information Association*, 11 (2004): 448–57.

12. V. Carpenter and B. Colwell, "Cancer Knowledge, Self-Efficacy, and Cancer Screening Behaviors among Mexican-American Women," *Journal of Cancer Education*, 10, 4 (1995): 217–22; cited in Tseng and Streltzer, *Cultural Competence in Health Care*, 27.

13. In this context, small talk is not Martin Heidegger's "idle talk," talk that is simply to fill in the silence and spaces of our being, talk that is ultimately meaningless.

14. Tseng and Streltzer, *Cultural Competence in Health Care*, 31.

15. A. H. Swota, "Cultural Diversity in the Clinical Setting," in *Ethics by Committee*, ed. D. Micah Hester (Lanham, MD: Rowman & Littlefield, 2008):117.

16. I discuss this in the context of Merleau-Ponty's notion of reversibility in Michael C. Brannigan, "Reversibility as a Radical Ground for an Ontology of the Body in Medicine," *Personalist Forum*, 8, 1 (1992): 219–24; see also my "Approaching an Ontology of the Body," *American Philosophical Association Newsletter on Philosophy and Medicine*, 89, 3 (Spring 1990), and "A Phenomenological Orientation to Illness and Ethical Implications," *Contemporary Philosophy*, 10, 8 (Spring 1985).

17. Tseng and Streltzer, *Cultural Competence in Health Care*, 37.

18. This section is adapted from my article, Michael C. Brannigan, "Presence in Suffering," 173–79.

19. For an instructive analysis, see Mei-Hui Tsai, *Opening Hearts and Minds: A Linguistic Framework for Analyzing Open Questions in Doctor-Patient Communication* (Taipei, Taiwan: Crane Publishing Company, 2006).

20. Elisabeth Macdonald, ed., *Difficult Conversations in Medicine* (Oxford: Oxford University Press, 2004): 6–7.

21. This is not to diminish the value of digital communication in certain instances. At the time of this writing, due to an unprecedented earthquake, tsunami, and nuclear meltdown, Japan suffers its worst national tragedy since World War II. For some time, I was only able to communicate with friends in Tokyo and elsewhere through digital means.

22. Max Picard, *The World of Silence*, trans. S. Godman (Washington, DC: Regnery Gateway, 1988).

23. Our addiction to speed is not just American. For instance, in Japan, Totenko restaurants charge their customers, not according to what they eat, but by the minute. There are over 100 of them in Japan. See James Gleick, *Faster: The Acceleration of Just About Everything* (New York: Vintage Books, Random House, 1999): 244.

24. Alan Lightman, "The World Is Too Much with Me," in *Living with the Genie: Essays on Technology and the Quest for Human Mastery*, ed. Alan Lightman, Daniel Sarawitz, and Christina Dresser (Washington, DC: Island Press, 2003): 287–303. In the 1950s, due to new time-saving technologies, experts predicted such increased efficiency and productivity that we would have a twenty-hour work week by 2000. Eleven years later, we are still waiting.

25. Some of the following ideas are adapted from one of my newspaper columns, Michael Brannigan, "Slow Down, Waste Time, Recharge," *Albany Times Union*, February 20, 2011; also online at http://www.timesunion.com/brannigan/.

26. Thomas Hylland Eriksen, *Tyranny of the Moment: Fast and Slow Time in the Information Age* (London: Pluto Press, 2001).

Appendix: Principles of Healthcare Ethics

For readers less familiar with what have become the standard moral principles in healthcare, here is a thumbnail sketch. As the main architects of these principles, Thomas Beauchamp and James Childress elaborate upon them in detail in their classic *Principles of Biomedical Ethics*. These principles have been further analyzed and commented on in numerous articles and books. The following shorthand approach does little justice to the intricacies of each principle. For a thorough exposition, see Beauchamp and Childress' comprehensive study.

AUTONOMY

Autonomy, from the Greek literally meaning "self-rule," is the now cherished principle of self-determination, considered by many to be the cornerstone in healthcare ethics. It underscores the notion that persons possess the fundamental moral right to make their own decisions regarding their well-being. In turn, each patient has the moral right to make healthcare decisions on his and her own behalf so that patient autonomy undergirds the patient's right to make an informed consent. Respecting a patient's informed consent is thus respecting a patient's autonomy. Autonomy has burgeoned as a moral principle especially in the past three decades and generated the movement regarding patients' rights, such as a patient's right to make end-of-life decisions including, for example, the right to request the withholding or withdrawal of life-sustaining treatment.

77

Philosophical grounds for self-determination derive from the view that persons are inherently moral agents and therein possess moral status. Here, Immanuel Kant's (1724–1804) ethical theory provides much of the conceptual backbone and highlights the idea of each person as a moral agent in that each person has the moral right to determine and set the course for his or her welfare. Personhood is thus associated with moral agency or moral status. Moral status refers to the possession of fundamental moral rights, and the exercise of moral rights rests upon the right to self-rule. Moreover, this right to self-determination is contingent upon certain conditions: one must be both free and competent to exercise self-rule. Freedom to exercise self-determination entails being free from coercion and from excessive manipulation. Though pressures and constraints always exist when making decisions, these in themselves do not preclude a free decision. Problems exist when such pressures become inordinate, disproportionate, and extreme. The proper exercise of moral agency, or autonomy, also presumes that the patient has sufficient decision-making capacity and is competent to make decisions. An incompetent patient does not lose the right to exercise autonomy. However, the incompetent patient cannot, as incompetent, exercise self-determination. For example, an advance directive is operative once a patient is no longer able to make decisions for himself. Yet in respecting a patient's advance directive, as a documented expression of a patient's autonomous choice, we are at the same time respecting his or her autonomy and moral agency. We are respecting the patient as a person. In the absence of an advance directive, efforts are made to ascertain what the patient would likely prefer and choose, a process that applies "substituted judgment." Even when there is little evidence to determine what a specific patient would decide, courts will refer to what "reasonable persons" in that similar situation would likely choose, applying a "best interests" principle.

Another key idea in Kant lies in his prohibition against viewing and treating persons merely as a means to an end. He persuasively argues against viewing persons merely as objects or instruments. Instead, he advocates that we view and treat all persons as ends-in-themselves, as subjects and thereby self-determining moral agents.

Bear in mind that having a moral right to self-determination is not equivalent to having a moral duty to self-determination. This may impose an unfair burden of decision-making upon patients who have become accustomed to the more traditional practice of deferring to their physicians' opinion and decision. Nonetheless, not assuming the role of primary decision-maker and relegating that role to the physician or others (as occurs in other cultures) is in itself an autonomous act as the patient still chooses in deciding not to choose.

Beauchamp and Childress elaborate further on the proactive nature of respecting a person's autonomy and moral agency:

To respect an autonomous agent is, at a minimum, to acknowledge that person's right to hold views, to make choices, and to take actions based on personal values and beliefs. Such respect involves respectful *action*, not merely a respectful *attitude*. It also requires more than noninterference in others' personal affairs. It includes, at least in some contexts, obligations to build up or maintain others' capacities for autonomous choice while helping to allay fears and other conditions that destroy or disrupt their autonomous actions. Respect, on this account, involves acknowledging decision-making rights and enabling persons to act autonomously, whereas disrespect for autonomy involves attitudes and actions that insult, ignore, or demean others' rights of autonomy.[1]

BENEFICENCE

A longstanding, esteemed principle in medical practice, beneficence literally means "doing good" or "making good" and refers to the physician's (and all health professionals') commitment to act in the best way capable in order to benefit the patient. This occurs on various levels such as working to improve the patient's health status, returning the patient to some level of normalcy as well as can be, enhancing the patient's welfare, sustaining the patient through a difficult ordeal, and preserving the patient's life.

Beneficence lies at the core of what it means to be a healthcare provider as a professional. Here, the importance of professionalism cannot be underestimated. As a professional, the physician is fully committed to act in the best interests of her patient, and in so doing embodies the moral fiber of her profession. Genuine professionalism in the healthcare setting requires a moral commitment to serve and work on the patient's behalf in the best way possible. One of the most thorough and engaging analyses of physician professionalism and its moral character lies in the work of Edmund Pellegrino. Moreover, he and David Thomasma, in their *For the Patient's Good: The Restoration of Beneficence in Health Care* insightfully underscore the role and importance of beneficence, particularly in view of the current climate in the U.S. that heralds patient autonomy, and as a consequence leads to occasional conflicts between the two principles of autonomy and beneficence. A typical case in which the principle of beneficence appears to conflict with the principle of autonomy occurs when a competent patient requests the removal of life-sustaining treatment such as a ventilator, knowing full well that this would lead to his death. He chooses to forego further treatment for various reasons: continued burden of treatment, emotional and financial burden on his family, and so on. His exercise of autonomy, however, may clash with his physician's sense of commitment to the patient in keeping with the principle of beneficence, acting in the patient's best interests through keeping him alive, alert, and able to communicate with family.

In our American socio-cultural milieu that espouses individualism and individual freedom, individual self-determination often prevails over considerations of beneficence. As we've seen in this text, this can also give way to cultural conflicts, for instance, when a patient represents a culture in which family decision-making, or family autonomy, prevails over individual patient decision-making, and yet we may still, as health providers, insist upon patient autonomy. The same culture that upholds family autonomy also tends to defer to the physician's authority in acting in the patient's best interests, congruent with beneficence.

Whether beneficence as commitment to the individual patient is unconditional presents another challenge since we must also consider the impact upon other patients as well as non-patients. Commitment to the single patient in view of respecting each patient as a person and as an end in himself complies with Kantian ethics. Yet the utilitarian ethics of John Stuart Mill (1806–1873) demands that we consider consequences upon others in light of what constitutes the greater good, even though maximizing the total good may seem counterintuitive to genuine fairness if it entails violating individual patients' rights.

As we will see in the case of nonmaleficence, there are some inherent challenges. First, what precisely is the scope of "benefit" regarding the patient's well-being? In the Hippocratic Oath the physician vows to benefit the patient, whereas benefit is more closely construed as the patient's health in the World Medical Association's Declaration of Geneva, adopted in Sept. 1948. How far does benefit extend, for instance, when the American Nurses Association 2001 code directs nursing care to address the patient's "health, well-being, and safety"?[2]

Along these lines, interpretive issues prevail as to the meaning of benefit, ranging from non-medical benefit (personal and relational such as finishing a manuscript, ironing out tensions with family, making it to a wedding anniversary, etc.) to more strictly medical determinations. Even among the latter, there are different levels of importance attached to medical treatments and their respective benefits (for example, chemotherapy in combination with radiation or chemotherapy alone or neither). In itself, the benefit of preserving life naturally conflicts with the benefit of sustaining life with some measure of qualitative communication with significant others. The question lies in how physicians themselves define their commitment to a patient's well-being. Along these lines, treatment that is determined to be medically futile (useless, or unable to attain its proper goal) may not be considered personally futile from the patient or family's perspective. And while there are varying levels of measurability with medical benefits, personal benefits are less measurable. Moreover, in the case of nonmaleficence, the value of alleviating or reducing suffering may clash with the value of preserving life.

A further problem arises particularly in the current climate of dwindling and scarce medical resources. Besides the patient, to what degree does the physician have an obligation to benefit others such as the patient's family (protecting a spouse from possible HIV infection while overriding patient confidentiality), the physician's family (protecting the family first during a disaster), the wider society (allocating ventilators during a pandemic), and even the physician's profession (going on strike to demand better working conditions at patients' expense, or refusing to violate professional standards of medical care at the patient's request, such as providing a lethal combination of drugs)?[3]

NONMALEFICENCE

Nonmaleficence is the other side of the coin of beneficence. In medical practice, the traditional maxim *primum non nocere* means "first do no harm" so that nonmaleficence denotes refraining from acting in ways that incur unnecessary pain and suffering to the patient. Along with beneficence, nonmaleficence remains a long-held and treasured principle throughout the history of Western medicine, and requires health professionals to avoid, prevent, minimize, and alleviate unnecessary harm to the patient. However, as with beneficence, problems occur due to varying interpretations of "nonharming."

One of the most plaguing problems healthcare providers face now and into the future is "physician-assisted suicide" (PAS). Countries such as the Netherlands and Luxembourg have legalized, or decriminalized, physician-assisted suicide under strict conditions. In similar fashion, Oregon has also passed referendums allowing for PAS. Does a physician who agrees to provide lethal medication for his patient at the patient's competent request violate the principle of nonmaleficence? He may act in a way that respects his patient's autonomy, but does he also at the same time act contrary to his patient's best interests, violating beneficence? Here nonmaleficence can mean either preventing the irrevocable harm of death, in which case the physician does violate the principle, or it could mean alleviating any further needless suffering on the part of the patient, in which case he acts in accord with the principle. Challenges exist when the duty to relieve harm conflicts with the duty to benefit the patient. How do we assess which principle has priority? There is no clear-cut rule. Usually, it is a matter of weighing benefits and burdens in specific instances. Yet even here, there is no hard and fast rule regarding what constitutes maximal benefits and burdens.

Of particular concern here is the matter of harm, for harm can wear various meanings. Usually, in the clinical setting, it refers to bodily and emotional injury and pain, suffering, disability, and death. In a broader sense, it also includes wrongs incurred upon the patient, often without him or her knowing this. Violating a patient's rights may be a type of harm. Beauchamp and Childress further point out that harm not only involves actual harm, but the real risk of serious harm while distinguishing between causal, legal, and moral responsibility and qualifying nonmaleficence with the "standard of due care":

> Obligations of nonmaleficence are not only obligations of not inflicting harms but also include obligations of not imposing *risks* of harm. A person can harm or place another person at risk without malicious or harmful intent, and the agent of harm may or may not be morally or legally responsible for the harms. In some cases, agents are causally responsible for a harm when they do not intend or are unaware of the harm caused . . .
>
> In cases of risk imposition, law and morality recognize a standard of due care that determines whether the agent who is causally responsible for the risk is legally or morally responsible as well. We can appropriately view this standard as a specification of the principle of nonmaleficence. Due care is taking sufficient and appropriate care to avoid causing harm, as the circumstances demand of a reasonable and prudent person. This standard requires that the goals pursued justify the risks that must be imposed to achieve these goals.[4]

The above discussion of autonomy, beneficence, and nonmaleficence reveals that no one principle is absolute. At the least, upholding these principles as absolute would be logically contradictory given the fact that they conflict with each other in certain circumstances. Ethical analysis must grapple with the challenging task of ascertaining which principle assumes priority in each situation. On account of our socio-cultural bias towards individual autonomy, this especially demands addressing the conflict evenhandedly. The non-absoluteness of these principles also reminds us that moral rights in themselves are not absolute. Thus having a moral right does not necessarily mean it is always right to exercise that same moral right in view of legitimate constraints, such as when the exercise of self-determination incurs harm to others.

JUSTICE

Justice has recently assumed a more prominent place among the four principles in view of increasing awareness of our limited healthcare resources in the face of escalating health demand. How do we fairly distribute healthcare resources? Also, the fact that a substantial portion of the U.S. remains uninsured brings the question of justice all the more to the table. These questions call for reasonable principles of fairness and equity.

Justice is perhaps the most complex of the principles. On its most basic level, according to Aristotle, it means treating equals equally, often referred to as the formal theory of justice. Yet Aristotle's depiction, as it stands, is clearly incomplete and lacks specificity. What are relevant moral differences that allow for unequal treatment, and what does being treated equally mean? There are differing theories of justice, further compounding notions of fairness, equality, and equity. Beauchamp and Childress classify justice theories as utilitarian (aiming to maximize the good), egalitarian (highlighting equal access for all), libertarian (emphasizing individual rights and fair process), and communitarian (emphasizing community tradition and practice).[5] In principle, the utilitarian approach appears sensible as it seeks to bring about overall collective long-term well-being. Conceptually rooted in Jeremy Bentham's (1748–1832) principle of utility (maximizing pleasure) and later John Stuart Mill's maximization of happiness or good, it would seem that justice theories necessarily incorporate the same aim of enhancing social well-being. However, what is meant by social well-being and whether various means to achieve this end are *per se* legitimate remain contentious issues and thus result in conflicting theories of justice.

In a communitarian view of justice, standards are derived from the community and its views regarding what constitutes the good life and the good society. For instance, Beauchamp and Childress cite the Netherlands' commitment to social solidarity in its prioritizing care for vulnerable populations of elderly and disabled.[6]

An egalitarian scheme underscores distributive justice. When applied to healthcare, distributive justice, in light of varying disparities and inequities, seeks to provide resources fairly so that those at the lowest end of the scale, the most poor and destitute and those without access to basic healthcare services, stand to gain from the sharing of resources. In addition, in emphasizing equal access to basic healthcare, distributive justice requires that we work in ways to ensure that the uninsured have such access. The most prolific proponent of distributive justice is John Rawls, who offers a thorough analysis in his classic *A Theory of Justice*. In his *Just Health Care*, Norman Daniels extends Rawls' analysis by proposing that healthcare resources be distributed in order for all to have fair equality of opportunity. Daniels' application of Rawls to healthcare underscores socioeconomic determinants that in turn impact on healthcare distribution.

In contrast, a libertarian approach to justice promotes more of an entitlement view of distributive justice, namely that a system is just when we each receive that which is due to us on account of what we each fairly and reasonably contribute. Persons are entitled to the fruits of their labors. Therefore, working to enable access to basic healthcare is virtuous, but cannot be demanded, otherwise it violates fundamental principles of fairness and entitlement. The foremost proponent here is Robert Nozick in his landmark *Anarchy, State, and Utopia*. For Nozick, distributive justice in a society occurs when individuals in that society are given what they are entitled to through reasonable acquisition and fair means. This clearly counters the egalitarian view of distributive justice espoused by Rawls. Nozick advocates the centrality of a free-market approach, thus focusing more on fair process than on outcomes. His entitlement theory of justice emphasizes the protection of individual rights, so that fair methods of acquiring, transferring, and rectifying are what make for fair process, and thus a fair society. As Beauchamp and Childress state:

> no pattern of just distribution exists independent of free-market procedures of
> acquiring property, legitimately transferring that property, and providing rec-
> tification for those whose property was illegitimately taken or who otherwise
> were illegitimately obstructed in the free market. [7]

To illustrate the complexity of justice theory, consider the question of allocating scarce resources during a pandemic. How do we fairly weigh the following criteria when deciding to whom we should allocate limited available antibiotics: medical need, queuing, ability to pay, social contribution, or age? Each criteria reflects some measure of how we view fairness for individual well-being and for the greater good. Should the primary criterion rest on medical need for those most in need of medical treatment? Yet those in dire need may not stand to gain from antibiotics as much as someone else who is less sick. Effective use of scarce resources may necessitate overriding the sickest patient. The crucial question remains—Who benefits the most from a medical treatment? A not uncommon scenario occurs when a health provider, at the insistence of patients, prescribes antibiotics for a viral infection, an infection which, unlike a bacterial infection, will still run its course with or without antibiotics. Overuse of antibiotics could result in producing a resistant bacteria strain, in turn possibly producing more serious infections later. [8] The idea that treatment ought to be provided on the basis of medical need carries assumptions as to the treatment's effectiveness for that specific patient. Is there an overriding duty to respect the patient's wish who insists on antibiotics for his viral infection?

As we see with all four principles, fundamental questions persist. Does medical treatment serve the patient's interest and well-being? Does it benefit the patient? Again, what constitutes benefit? And what about non-medical, personal benefits? Our challenge lies not only in reasonably evaluating the role of these principles in healthcare settings, but in assessing their force in view of cultural differences and fault lines we've discussed albeit briefly in this work.

NOTES

1. Tom L. Beauchamp and James F. Childress, *Principles of Biomedical Ethics*, 5th ed. (New York: Oxford University Press, 2011): 63.

2. Robert M. Veatch, Amy M. Haddad, and Dan C. English, *Case Studies in Biomedical Ethics: Decision-Making, Principles, and Cases* (New York: Oxford University Press, 2010): 73.

3. Veatch, *Case Studies*, 85–95.

4. Beauchamp and Childress, *Principles of Biomedical Ethics*, 117–18.

5. Beauchamp and Childress, *Principles of Biomedical Ethics*, 230ff.

6. Beauchamp and Childress, *Principles of Biomedical Ethics*, 233.

7. Beauchamp and Childress, *Principles of Biomedical Ethics*, 232.

8. Veatch, *Case Studies*, 103–4.

Bibliography

Akabayashi, Akira, Satoshi Kodama, and B.T. Slingsby. *Biomedical Ethics in Asia: A Casebook for Multicultural Learners*. Singapore: McGraw-Hill, 2010.

Andrulis, Dennis, Thomas Delbianco, Laura Avakian, and Yoku Shaw-Taylor. *Conducting a Cultural Competence Self-Assessment*. http://www.consumerstar.org/pubs/Culturalcompselfassess.pdf.

Appiah, Kwame Anthony. *The Ethics of Identity*. Princeton, NJ: Princeton University Press, 2005.

———. *Cosmpolitanism: Ethics in a World of Strangers*. New York: Norton, 2006.

Balint, John. "Rethinking the Social Role of Physicians: The Importance of Physicians' 'Symbolic Acts.'" NYSBA *Health Law Journal* 11, no. 3 (Summer/Fall 2006): 54–59.

Balint, Michael. *The Doctor, the Patient, and the Illness*. London: Tavistock Publications, 1957.

Bauman, Zygmunt. *Globalization: The Human Consequences*. New York: Columbia University Press, 1998.

———. Trans. (from Polish) by Lydia Bauman. *Culture in a Liquid Modern World*. Cambridge, UK: Polity, 2011.

Beauchamp, Thomas, and James Childress. *Principles of Biomedical Ethics*. 5th ed. New York: Oxford University Press, 2011.

Betancourt, J.R., A.R. Green, and J.E. Carrillo. *Cultural Competence in Health Care: Emerging Frameworks and Practical Approaches*. New York: Commonwealth Fund, 2002.

Blank, Robert H., and Janna C. Merrick, eds. *End-of-Life Decision Making: A Cross-National Study*. Cambridge, MA: MIT Press, 2005.

Brannigan, Michael C. "Reversibility as a Radical Ground for an Ontology of the Body in Medicine." *Personalist Forum* 8, no.1 (1992): 219–24.

———. "A Chronicle of Organ Transplant Progress in Japan," *Transplant International* 5 (1992): 180–86.

———. "Designing Ethicists." *Health Care Analysis* 4 (1996): 206–18.

———. "Connecting the Dots in Cultural Competency: Institutional Strategies and Conceptual Caveats." *Cambridge Quarterly of Healthcare Ethics* 17 (2008):173–84.

———. "*Ikiru* and Net-Casting in Intercultural Bioethics," pp. 345–65 in *Bioethics at the Movies*, edited by Sandra Shapshay. Baltimore, MD: The Johns Hopkins University Press, 2009.

———. "Presence in Suffering: Lessons from the Buddhist Four Noble Truths." *Eubios Journal of Asian and International Bioethics* 20 (November 2010): 173–79.

Brannigan, Michael C., and Judith A. Boss. *Healthcare Ethics in a Diverse Society*. Mountain View, CA: Mayfield Pub. Co., 2001.

Brecker, Bob. *Torture and the Ticking Bomb*. Malden, MA: Blackwell Publishing, 2007.

Campinha-Bacote, Josepha. *The Process of Cultural Competence in Health Care: A Culturally Competent Model of Care*. 2nd ed. Wyoming, OH: Transcultural C.A.R.E. Associates, 1994.

Carpenter, V., and B. Colwell. "Cancer Knowledge, Self-Efficacy, and Cancer Screening Behaviors among Mexican-American Women." *Journal of Cancer Education* 10, no. 4 (1995): 217–22.

Chang, Betty L., Suzanne Bakken, S. Scott Brown, Thomas K. Houston, Gary L. Kreps, Rita Kukafka, Charles Safran, and Zoe Stavri. "Bridging the Digital Divide: Reaching Vulnerable Populations." *Journal of the American Medical Information Association* 11 (2004): 448–57.

Cioffi, J. "Nurses Experiences of Caring for Culturally Diverse Patients in an Acute Care Setting." *Contemporary Nurse* 20 (2005): 78–86.

Cohen, Richard. "Introduction: Humanism and Anti-Humanism—Levinas, Cassirer, and Heidegger," pp. vii–xliv in Emmanuel Levinas, *Humanism of the Other*, trans. Nidra Poller. Urbana: University of Illinois Press, 2006.

Cohen, Stanley. *States of Denial: Knowing about Atrocities and Suffering*. Cambridge, UK: Polity, 2001.

Coward, Harold, and Pinit Ratanakul, eds. *A Cross-Cultural Dialogue on Health Care Ethics*. Waterloo, Ontario: Wilfred Laurier University Press, 1999.

Crigger, Nancy, Michael Brannigan, and Martha Baird. "Compassionate Nursing Professionals as Good Citizens of the World." *Advances in Nursing Science* 29, no.1 (January 2006): 15–26.

Crigger, Nancy, and Lygia Holcomb. "Practical Strategies for Providing Culturally Sensitive, Ethical Care in Developing Nations." *Journal of Transcultural Nursing* 18, no.1 (January 2007): 70–76.

Daniels, Norman. *Just Health Care*. New York: Cambridge University Press, 1985.

DasGupta, Sayantani. "Narrative Humility." *Lancet* 371 (March 22, 2008): 980–81.

Eckenwiler, Lisa A., and Felicia G. Cohn, eds. *The Ethics of Bioethics: Mapping the Moral Landscape*. Baltimore, MD: The Johns Hopkins University Press, 2007.

Ekintumas, D. "Nursing in Thailand: Western Concepts vs. Thai Tradition." *International Nursing Review* 46 (1999): 55–57.

Elliott, Carl. *Better than Well: American Medicine Meets the American Dream*. New York: Norton, 2003.

Englehardt, H. Tristram, Jr., ed. *Global Bioethics: The Collapse of Consensus*. Salem, MA: M&M Scrivener Press, 2006.

Eriksen, Thomas Hylland. *Tyranny of the Moment: Fast and Slow Time in the Information Age*. London: Pluto Press, 2001.

Farmer, Paul. *Pathologies of Power: Health, Human Rights, and the New War on the Poor*. Berkeley: University of California Press, 2003.

———. "Blog from the Mountains of Northern Rwanda." Team Heart Text. http://teamheart-text.blogspot.com/ (22 Feb. 2011).

Fox, Renée C. *The Sociology of Medicine: A Participant Observer's View*. Englewood Cliffs, NJ: Prentice Hall, 1989.

———. "The Entry of U.S. Bioethics into the 1990s: A Sociological Analysis," pp. 21–71 in *A Matter of Principles? Ferment in U.S. Bioethics*, edited by E.R. Du Bose, R. Hamel, and L.J. O'Connell. Valley Forge, PA: Trinity Press International, 1994.

———. "Khayelitsha Journal." *Society* 42, no. 4 (May/June 2005): 70–76.

Fox, Renée C., and Judith P. Swazey. *Spare Parts: Organ Replacement in American Society*. New York: Oxford University Press, 1992.

———. "Examining American Bioethics: Its Problems and Prospects. Quo Vadis?" *Cambridge Quarterly of Health Care Ethics* 14 (2005): 361–73.

———. *Observing Bioethics*. Oxford: Oxford University Press, 2008.

Galanti, Geri-Ann. *Caring for Patients from Different Cultures: Case Studies from American Hospitals*. 2nd ed. Philadelphia: University of Pennsylvania Press, 1997.

Geertz, Clifford. *The Interpretation of Cultures*. New York: Basic Books, 1973.

————. *Available Light: Anthropological Reflections on Philosophical Topics*. Princeton, NJ: Princeton University Press, 2000.

Gleick, James. *Faster: The Acceleration of Just About Everything*. New York: Vintage Books, Random House, 1999.

Gordon, Elisa J. "Bioethics: Contemporary Anthropological Approaches," pp. 73–86 in *Encyclopedia of Medical Anthropology: Health and Illness in the World's Cultures*, edited by Carol R. Ember and Melvin Ember. Dordrecht: Kluwer/Plenum Publishers, 2004.

————. "Health & Disease: III. Anthropological Perspectives," pp. 1070–75 in *Encyclopedia of Bioethics*, 3rd ed., edited by Stephen G. Post. New York: Macmillan Reference, 2004.

Gowans, Christopher W., ed. *Moral Dilemmas*. New York: Oxford University Press, 1987.

Hahn, Robert A. *Sickness and Healing: An Anthropological Perspective*. New Haven: Yale University Press, 1995.

Herman, Barbara. "Pluralism and the Community of Moral Judgment," pp. 60–80 in *Toleration: An Elusive Virtue*, edited by David Heyd. Princeton, NJ: Princeton University Press, 1996.

Heschel, Abraham J. *The Insecurity of Freedom*. New York: Noonday Press, 1966.

Horton, John. "Toleration as a Virtue," pp. 28–43 in *Toleration: An Elusive Virtue*, edited by David Heyd. Princeton, NJ: Princeton University Press, 1996.

Iacoboni, Marco. *Mirroring People: The Science of Empathy and How We Connect with Others*. New York: Picador/Farrar, Straus and Giroux, 2008.

Jeffreys, Marianne R. *Teaching Cultural Competence in Nursing and Health Care: Inquiry, Action, and Innovation*. New York: Springer, 2006.

Kant, Immanuel. "Introduction to the Metaphysic of Morals." In *The Doctrine of Virtue, Part II of the Metaphysic of Morals*, translated by Mary J. Gregory. Philadelphia: University of Pennsylvania Press, 1971.

Kass, Leon R. "The Wisdom of Repugnance." *New Republic* 216, no. 22 (June 2, 1997): 17–26.

Kim, Min-Sun. *Non-Western Perspectives on Human Communication: Implications for Theory and Practice*. Thousand Oaks, CA: Sage Publications, 2002.

Kleinman, Arthur. *Patients and Healers in the Context of Culture: Exploration of the Borderland between Anthropology, Medicine, and Psychiatry*. Berkeley: University of California Press, 1980.

————. *The Illness Narratives: Suffering, Healing, and the Human Condition*. New York: Basic Books, 1988.

————. *Social Origins of Distress and Disease: Depression, Neurasthenia, and Pain in Modern China*. New Haven: Yale University Press, 1988.

————. *Writing at the Margin: Discourse Between Anthropology and Medicine*. Berkeley: University of California Press, 1995.

Kosoko-Lasaki, Sade, Cynthia T. Cook, and Richard L. O'Brien, eds. *Cultural Proficiency in Addressing Health Disparities*. Sudbury, MA: Jones and Bartlett Publishers, 2009.

Kulwicki, Anahid Dervartanian. "People of Arab Heritage," pp. 90–105 in *Transcultural Health Care: A Culturally Competent Approach*, 2nd ed., edited by Larry D. Purnell and Betty J. Paulanka. Philadelphia: F.A. Davis Company, 2003.

Leininger, M., and M.R. MacFarland, eds. *Transcultural Nursing: Concepts, Theories, Research and Practice*. 3rd ed. New York: McGraw-Hill, 2002.

Levinas, Emmanuel. *Totality and Infinity*, translated by Alphonso Lingis. Pittsburgh, PA: Duquesne University Press, 1969.

————. *Existence and Existents*, translated by Alphonso Lingis. The Hague and Boston: Martinus Nijhoff, 1978.

————. *Otherwise than Being: Or Beyond Essence*, translated by Alphonso Lingis. Pittsburgh, PA: Duquesne University Press, 1981.

————. *Ethics and Infinity: Conversations with Philippe Nemo*, translated by Richard A. Cohen. Pittsburgh, PA: Duquesne University Press, 1985.

————. *Time and the Other*, translated by Richard A. Cohen. Pittsburgh, PA: Duquesne University Press, 1987.

————. *Alterity and Transcendence*, translated by Michael B. Smith. New York: Columbia University Press, 1999.

————. *Humanism of the Other*, translated Nidra Poller. Urbana: University of Illinois Press, 2006.

Lightman, Alan. "The World Is Too Much with Me," pp. 287–303 in *Living with the Genie: Essays on Technology and the Quest for Human Mastery*, edited by Alan Lightman, Daniel Sarawitz, and Christina Dresser. Washington, DC: Island Press, 2003.

Lock, Margaret. *Twice Dead: Organ Transplants and the Reinvention of Death*. Berkeley: University of California Press, 2002.

Lumetra. *The Cultural Competence Self-Assessment Protocol for Managed Care Organizations*; *Developing a Self-Assessment Tool for Culturally and Linguistically Appropriate Services in Local Public Health Agencies: Final Report*. Rockville, MD: U.S. DHHS, 2003.

Macdonald, Elisabeth, ed. *Difficult Conversations in Medicine*. Oxford: Oxford University Press, 2004.

Macer, Darryl. "End of Life Care in Japan," pp. 110–29 in *End-of-Life Decision Making: A Cross-National Study*, edited by Robert H. Blank and Janna C. Merrick. Cambridge, MA: MIT Press, 2005.

Macklin, Ruth. "Ethical Relativism in a Multicultural Society." *Kennedy Institute of Ethics Journal* 8, no.1 (1998): 1–22.

————. *Against Relativism: Cultural Diversity and the Search for Ethical Universals in Medicine*. New York: Oxford University Press, 1999.

Marcus, Ruth Barcan. "Moral Dilemmas and Consistency," pp. 188–204 in *Moral Dilemmas*, edited by Christopher W. Gowans. New York: Oxford University Press, 1987.

Marshall, Patricia A., and Barbara A. Koenig. "Accounting for Culture in a Globalized Bioethics." *Journal of Law, Medicine & Ethics* 32, no. 2 (2004): 252–56.

————. "Anthropology and Bioethics," pp. 215–25, Vol. 1 in *Encyclopedia of Bioethics*, 3rd ed., edited by Stephen G. Post. New York: Gale Group/Macmillan, 2004.

Meleis, A.I., and A. Jonsen. "Ethical Crises and Cultural Differences." *Western Journal of Medicine* 138, no. 6 (June 1983): 889–892.

Minnesota Department of Human Services. *Guidelines for Culturally Competent Organizations*. 2nd ed., http://www.leg.state.mn.us/docs/2005/other/050050.pdf (May 2004).

National Center for Cultural Competence, Georgetown University Child Development Center. http://www.georgetown.edu/research/gucdc/nccc/ncccorgselfassess.pdf.

Nicholson, Peter. "Toleration as Moral Ideal," pp. 158–73 in *Aspects of Toleration: Philosophical Studies*, edited by John Horton and Susan Mendus. London: Methuen, 1985.

Noddings, Nel. *Caring: A Feminine Approach to Ethics and Moral Education*. 2nd ed. Berkeley: University of California Press, 1984.

Nordstrom, Carolyn. "Fault Lines," pp. 63–87 in *Global Health in Times of Violence*, edited by Barbara Rylko-Bauer, Linda Whiteford, and Paul Farmer. Santa Fe, NM: School for Advanced Research Press, 2009.

Nozick, Robert. *Anarchy, State, and Utopia*. New York: Basic Books, 1974.

Ohnuki-Tierney, Emiko. *Kamikaze, Cherry Blossoms, and Nationalism: The Militarization of Aesthetics in Japanese History*. Chicago: University of Chicago Press, 2002.

O'Neill, Onora. *Autonomy and Trust in Bioethics*. Cambridge: Cambridge University Press, 2002.

Orfali K., and E.J. Gordon. "Autonomy Gone Awry: A Cross-Cultural Study of Parents' Experiences in Neonatal Intensive Care Units." *Theoretical Medicine and Bioethics* 25, no. 4 (2004): 329–365.

Payer, Lynn. *Medicine and Culture*. New York: Henry Holt, 1988.

Pellegrino, Edmund D. "Toward a Reconstruction of Medical Morality: The Primacy of the Act of Profession and the Fact of Illness." *Journal of Medicine and Philosophy* 4 (March 1979): 32–56.

————. "The Commodification of Medical and Health Care: The Moral Consequences of a Paradigm Shift from a Professional to a Market Ethic." *Journal of Medicine and Philosophy* 24 (1999): 243–266.

Pellegrino, Edmund D., and David C. Thomasma. *For the Patient's Good: The Restoration of Beneficence in Health Care*. New York: Oxford University Press, 1987.

————. *The Virtues in Medical Practice*. New York: Oxford University Press, 1993.

Perez, Miguel A., and Raffy R. Luquis, eds. *Cultural Competence in Health Education and Health Promotion.* San Francisco: Jossey-Bass, 2008.

Picard, Max. *The World of Silence*, translated by S. Godman. Washington, DC: Regnery Gateway, 1988.

Prograis, Lawrence J., Jr., and Edmund D. Pellegrino. *African American Bioethics: Culture, Race, and Identity.* Washington, DC: Georgetown University Press, 2007.

Purnell, Larry D., and Betty J. Paulanka, eds. *Transcultural Health Care: A Culturally Competent Approach.* 2nd ed. Philadelphia: F.A. Davis Company, 2003.

———. *Guide to Culturally Competent Health Care.* 2nd ed. Philadelphia: F.A. Davis Company, 2008.

Rawls, John. *A Theory of Justice.* Cambridge, MA: Belknap Press, Harvard University Press, 1971.

———. *The Law of Peoples.* Cambridge, MA: Harvard University Press, 1999.

Read, Margaret. *Culture, Health and Disease: Social and Cultural Influences on Health Programmes in Developing Countries.* London: Tavistock, 1966.

Ricoeur, Paul, ed. *Tolerance between Intolerance and the Intolerable.* Providence, RI: Berghahn Books, 1996.

Rylko-Bauer, Barbara, Linda Whiteford, and Paul Farmer, eds. *Global Health in Times of Violence.* Santa Fe, NM: School for Advanced Research Press, 2009.

Sarangi, Srikant, and Celia Roberts, eds. *Talk, Work and Institutional Order: Discourse on Medical, Mediation and Management Settings.* Berlin: Mouton de Gruyter, 1999.

Sartre, Jean-Paul. *No Exit and Three Other Plays.* New York: Random House, Vintage International, 1989.

Selekman, Janice. "People of Jewish Heritage," pp. 234–248 in *Transcultural Health Care: A Culturally Competent Approach.* 2nd ed., edited by Larry D. Purnell and Betty J. Paulanka. Philadelphia: F.A. Davis Company, 2003.

Shelton, Wayne, and Dyrleif Bjarnadottir. "Ethics Consultation and the Committee," pp. 49–77 in *Ethics by Committee: A Textbook on Consultation, Organization, and Education for Hospital Ethics Committees*, edited by D. Micah Hester. Lanham, MD: Rowman & Littlefield, 2008.

Shweder, Richard A. *Thinking Through Cultures: Expeditions in Cultural Psychology.* Cambridge, MA: Harvard University Press, 1991.

Smedley, Brian D., Adrienne Y. Stith, and Alan R. Nelson, eds. *Unequal Treatment: Confronting Racial and Ethnic Disparities in Health Care.* Washington, DC: The National Academies Press, Institute of Medicine of the National Academies, 2002.

Sontag, Susan. *Regarding the Pain of Others.* New York: Picador/Farrar, Straus and Giroux, 2003.

Spencer-Oatey, Helen, ed. *Culturally Speaking: Managing Rapport through Talk Across Cultures.* London: Continuum, 2000.

Surbone, Antonella. "Cultural Aspects of Communication in Cancer Care." *Recent Results in Cancer Research* 168 (2006): 91–104.

Swota, Alissa Hurwitz. "Cultural Diversity in the Clinical Setting," pp. 107–32 in *Ethics by Committee: A Textbook on Consultation, Organization, and Education for Hospital Ethics Committees*, edited by D. Micah Hester. Lanham, MD: Rowman & Littlefield, 2008.

ten Have, Henk. "Principlism: A Western European Appraisal," pp. 101–20 in *A Matter of Principles? Ferment in U.S. Bioethics*, edited by E.R. Du Bose, R. Hamel, and L.J. O'Connell. Valley Forge, PA: Trinity Press International, 1994.

ten Have, Henk, and Bert Gordijn, eds. *Bioethics in a European Perspective.* Dordrecht: Kluwer Academic Publishers, 2001.

Tervalon, Melanie, and Jann Murray-García. "Cultural Humility Versus Cultural Competence: A Critical Distinction in Defining Physician Training Outcomes in Multicultural Education." *Journal of Health Care for the Poor and Underserved* 9, no. 2 (May 1998): 117–25.

Tindale, Christopher. "The Logic of Torture." *Social Theory and Practice* 22 (1996): 349–74.

Truog, Robert D. "Tackling Medical Futility in Texas." *The New England Journal of Medicine* 357, no. 1 (July 5, 2007): 1–3.

Tsai, Mei-Hui. *Opening Hearts and Minds: A Linguistic Framework for Analyzing Open Questions in Doctor-Patient Communication*. Taipei, Taiwan: Crane Publishing Company, 2006.

Tseng, Wen-Shing, and Jon Streltzer. *Cultural Competence in Health Care: A Guide for Professionals*. New York: Springer, 2008.

Turkle, Sherry. *Alone Together: Why We Expect More from Technology and Less from Each Other*. New York: Basic Books, 2011.

Turner, Leigh. "Zones of Consensus and Zones of Conflict: Questioning the 'Common Morality' Presumption in Bioethics." *Kennedy Institute of Ethics Journal* 13, no. 3 (2003): 193–218.

Veatch, Robert M., Amy M. Haddad, and Dan C. English. *Case Studies in Biomedical Ethics: Decision-Making, Principles, and Cases*. New York, Oxford University Press, 2010.

Walden, George. *The New Elites: Making a Career in the Masses*. London: Allen Lane, Penguin Press, 2000.

Watsuji, Tetsuro. *Rinrigaku* (The Study of Ethics), trans. Yamamoto Seisaku. Albany: State University of New York Press, 1996; originally Tokyo: Iwanami Shoten Publishers, 1937.

Williams, Bernard. "Toleration: An Impossible Virtue?" pp. 18–27 in *Toleration: An Elusive Virtue*, edited by David Heyd. Princeton, NJ: Princeton University Press, 1996.

Wyschogrod, Edith. *Emmanuel Levinas: The Problem of Ethical Metaphysics*. 2nd ed. New York: Fordham University Press, 2000.

Index

time: and embodying presence, 74–75; perceptions/misconceptions about, 73; and temporal dimension of cultural competency, 20–21; time pressures/ constraints, 73, 74

tolerance: absolute/excessive, limits of, 48, 50; combining disapproval and restraint, 49–50; and context-sensitive judgments, 49; importance of context, 48; impossibility of, debates about, 48; of intolerable behaviors, xii, xiii, 50; limits of, challenges of determining, xii, 10, 48, 50, 69; and moral pluralism, 47; as non-intervention, 48; as philosophical concept, 47

tools and devices. *See* technology

torture, 41

tradition: modern vs., 38; reification of, 38; unfamiliar, defamation of, 48

translators, interpreters vs., 68

Tseng, Wen-Shing, 18, 22, 68

Turkish Muslims, care traditions, 6

Turner, Leigh, xii

Tuskegee trials, 7

Twice Dead: Organ Transplants and the Reinvention of Death (Lock), 22

underinsured/uninsured, 17

Uniform Determination of Death Act, 1981 (U.S.), 22

United Nations Educational, Scientific, and Cultural Organization's (UNESCO) 2005 Declaration on Bioethics and Human Rights, 23

United States: being-for-oneself vs. being-for-the-other, 54; organ transplants in, 22; personal isolation in, 35. *See also* healthcare delivery system; Western biomedicine

"Universal Declaration on Cultural Diversity" (UNESCO), 49

universal principles, assumptions about, 35–36, 47

utilitarian theory: arguments favoring torture, 41; conflicts between autonomy and beneficence, 80; justice, 83

values: culturally specific, xiii, 3, 5; fact/ value relationship, 29; socio-cultural assumptions about, 29. *See also* bioethics; morals/moral behavior

Vietnamese/Vietnamese traditions: attitudes about death, 6; importance of *bomoh*, 10

virtual personas, moral issues, 60n18

visage, face, and accountability to the Other, xii, 54

Vishnu, 56

voodoo medicine, 26

Walden, George, 64

Watsuki Tetsuro, 4

Western biomedicine: and assumptions about shared morality, xii, 10–11, 12; commoditization of patients, 39–40; and concept autonomy, 10, 34; and concepts of disease, 9; crisis orientation, 11; cultivating presence, challenges, 73; dominance of as worldview, xi, xii, 9, 36; focus on symptoms and cures, 11, 28; individualization of illness, 10; language of organic affliction, 10; measurability bias, 39–40; and mind-body dichotomy, 3; as one of many worldviews, 9, 12; organ transplants, 22, 29; physician authority, 26; secularized nature, 23; treatment approaches, 10. *See also* death; healthcare delivery system; morality; technology

Williams, Bernard, 48

World Medical Association's Declaration of Geneva, 80

worldview: assumptions about universality of, 23; clashes between, xiii, 3; cultural determinants, 4, 5; definition, 3; impact on healthcare decisions, 8, 29; and Western biomedicine, 9, 36

Wyschogrod, Edith, 54

Yahay Mohammed, 2

Yang, Foua (Hmong refugee), xi

About the Author

Michael C. Brannigan (Ph.D., Philosophy, M.A., Religious Studies, University of Leuven, Belgium) is the George and Jane Pfaff Endowed Chair in Ethics and Moral Values at The College of Saint Rose in Albany, New York. Holder of the first endowed chair in the college's history, he is also on the faculty of the Alden March Bioethics Institute at Albany Medical College. Prior to his appointment, he was vice president for Clinical and Organizational Ethics at the Center for Practical Bioethics in Kansas City, Missouri. Before that, he was founder and executive director of the Institute for Cross-Cultural Ethics at La Roche College, Pittsburgh, Pennsylvania.

To complement his rich and long-standing clinical experience as an ethics consultant, hospital ethics committee advisor, and hospice volunteer, his specialties lie in ethics, Asian philosophy, medical ethics, and intercultural ethics. Along with numerous articles, his books include *Ethics Across Cultures*; *Striking a Balance: A Primer in Traditional Asian Values*; *The Pulse of Wisdom: The Philosophies of India, China, and Japan*; *Healthcare Ethics in a Diverse Society* (co-authored); *Cross-Cultural Biotechnology*; and *Ethical Issues in Human Cloning*. He serves on the editorial boards of *Health Care Analysis: An International Journal of Health Care Philosophy and Policy* and *Communication and Medicine*. He also writes a monthly column on ethics for the *Albany Times Union*, at www.timesunion.com/brannigan/.

Michael was born in Fukuoka, Japan, as Kenji Kimura. He and his beautiful wife, Brooke, along with their dog, Seamus, live in Niskayuna, New York. For fun, he plays piano and tennis, ocean kayaks, and practices martial arts.